# INSOMNIA
## Don't Lose Sleep Over It

*Don't Lose Sleep Over It*

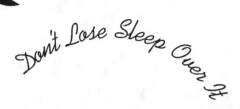

# INSOMNIA
## Finding the Help You Need

## Linda K. DeVries

Harold Shaw Publishers
Wheaton, Illinois

ISBN 0-87788-184-7

Cover and inside design by David LaPlaca
Cover illustration © 1998 by David LaPlaca

*Library of Congress Cataloging-in-Publication Data*

DeVries, Linda K
   Insomnia : don't lose sleep over it, find the help you need / by
Linda K. DeVries.
     p.  cm.
   Includes bibliographical references and index.
   ISBN 0-87788-184-7
    1. Insomnia—Popular works.    I. Title
RC548.D48
816.8′498—DC21                                                              97-50626
                                                                            CIP

03  02  01  00  99  98

10  9  8  7  6  5  4  3  2  1

To my husband, Dick,
and my daughters, Taryn and Jill,
with all my heart.

# Contents

Acknowledgments . . . . . . . . . . . . . . . . . . . . . . . . 11
Introduction . . . . . . . . . . . . . . . . . . . . . . . . . . 13

**1 Understanding Your Sleep Connection** . . . . . . . 15
    What Is Sleep? . . . . . . . . . . . . . . . . . . . . 16
    Effects of Too Little Sleep . . . . . . . . . . . . . 19
    Sleep Deprived? . . . . . . . . . . . . . . . . . . . 20
    How Much Sleep Do I Need? . . . . . . . . . . . . 21
    Sleep Needs Change with Age . . . . . . . . . . . 22

**2 Fixing a Faulty Sleep Connection** . . . . . . . . . . 24
    Causes of Insomnia . . . . . . . . . . . . . . . . . 24
    Types of Insomnia . . . . . . . . . . . . . . . . . . 25
    Charting Your Sleep History . . . . . . . . . . . . 27
    Keep a Sleep Journal . . . . . . . . . . . . . . . . 28
    Explore Your Life for Clues . . . . . . . . . . . . 29
    Physical Factors . . . . . . . . . . . . . . . . . . . 30
    Emotional Issues . . . . . . . . . . . . . . . . . . . 32
    Balanced Lifestyle . . . . . . . . . . . . . . . . . . 34

**3 The Mental Connection: Changing Your Attitudes
about Sleeplessness** . . . . . . . . . . . . . . . . . . 37
    You're Not Alone . . . . . . . . . . . . . . . . . . . 38
    Don't Try So Hard . . . . . . . . . . . . . . . . . . 39
    Avoid "Fear of Insomnia" . . . . . . . . . . . . . 41
    Correct Your Misperceptions . . . . . . . . . . . . 43
    Putting Your Brain to Bed . . . . . . . . . . . . . 43
    Don't Play the Victim . . . . . . . . . . . . . . . . 45
    Attitude Adjustment . . . . . . . . . . . . . . . . . 45

**4 The Physical Connection, Part 1: Checking for Medical Causes** . . . . . . . . . . . . . . . . . . . . . 47
    Gender Differences . . . . . . . . . . . . . . . . . . 48
    Sleep Patterns and Older Adults . . . . . . . . . . 50
    Pain, Illness, and Insomnia . . . . . . . . . . 51
    Power in Weakness . . . . . . . . . . . . . . . . 53
    Allergies . . . . . . . . . . . . . . . . . . . . . . 54
    Asthma . . . . . . . . . . . . . . . . . . . . . . 55

**5 The Physical Connection, Part 2: Understanding Sleep Disorders** . . . . . . . . . . . . . . . . . . . . 57
    Sleep Apnea . . . . . . . . . . . . . . . . . . . . 57
    Symptoms of Sleep Apnea . . . . . . . . . . . . 59
    Snoring . . . . . . . . . . . . . . . . . . . . . . 61
    Restless Legs Syndrome . . . . . . . . . . . . . 62
    Periodic Limb Movement . . . . . . . . . . . . . 64
    Nocturnal Leg Cramps . . . . . . . . . . . . . . 65
    Sleepwalking . . . . . . . . . . . . . . . . . . . 66
    REM-Sleep Behavior Disorder . . . . . . . . . . 67
    Tooth Grinding . . . . . . . . . . . . . . . . . . 67
    Narcolepsy . . . . . . . . . . . . . . . . . . . . 68

**6 The Behavioral Connection: Adjusting Your Lifestyle** . . . . . . . . . . . . . . . . . . . . . . . . 71
    Exercise . . . . . . . . . . . . . . . . . . . . . . 71
    Relax . . . . . . . . . . . . . . . . . . . . . . . . 72
    Take a Bath . . . . . . . . . . . . . . . . . . . . 74
    Try a Massage . . . . . . . . . . . . . . . . . . 76
    Watch Your Diet . . . . . . . . . . . . . . . . . 77
    Cut Out Caffeine . . . . . . . . . . . . . . . . . 79
    Avoid Alcohol . . . . . . . . . . . . . . . . . . 80
    Stop Smoking . . . . . . . . . . . . . . . . . . 80
    Bring Order to Your Day . . . . . . . . . . . . 81
    Do Something for Someone Else . . . . . . . . 82

**7 The Day-Night Connection: Resetting Your Internal Clock** . . . . . . . . . . . . . . . . . . . . 84
    Circadian Rhythms . . . . . . . . . . . . . . . 84
    The Nap Controversy . . . . . . . . . . . . . . 86
    Mood Swings . . . . . . . . . . . . . . . . . . 87
    Sunday-Night Insomnia . . . . . . . . . . . . 88
    Jet Lag . . . . . . . . . . . . . . . . . . . . . . 88

Shift Work . . . . . . . . . . . . . . . . . . . . . . . 90
Delayed Sleep Phase Syndrome . . . . . . . . . . . 92
Advanced Sleep Phase Syndrome . . . . . . . . . 92
Treating Circadian Phase Disorders . . . . . . . . 93

**8 The Environmental Connection: Setting the**
**Stage for Sleep** . . . . . . . . . . . . . . . . . . . . 95
Guard Your Bedroom . . . . . . . . . . . . . . . . 95
The Bed Factor . . . . . . . . . . . . . . . . . . . . 96
Steady Room Temperature . . . . . . . . . . . . . 98
Dim the Lights . . . . . . . . . . . . . . . . . . . . 99
Drown Out Noise . . . . . . . . . . . . . . . . . . . 99
The Clock . . . . . . . . . . . . . . . . . . . . . . . 100
Safe and Secure . . . . . . . . . . . . . . . . . . . 101
When You're Away from Home . . . . . . . . . . 101

**9 The Psychological Connection: Insomnia's**
**Emotional Causes** . . . . . . . . . . . . . . . . . . . 104
Worry and Anxiety . . . . . . . . . . . . . . . . . 105
Fear . . . . . . . . . . . . . . . . . . . . . . . . . . 106
Grief . . . . . . . . . . . . . . . . . . . . . . . . . . 108
Depression . . . . . . . . . . . . . . . . . . . . . . 109
Anger . . . . . . . . . . . . . . . . . . . . . . . . . 110

**10 The Spiritual Connection: Finding Rest for**
**the Soul** . . . . . . . . . . . . . . . . . . . . . . . . 112
A New Perspective . . . . . . . . . . . . . . . . . 113
Learning to Trust . . . . . . . . . . . . . . . . . . 114
Discovering God's Presence in Prayer . . . . . . 115
Reading the Bible for Encouragement . . . . . . 116

**11 The Family Connection: Your Child's**
**Sleep Needs** . . . . . . . . . . . . . . . . . . . . . . 118
Infants and Sleep . . . . . . . . . . . . . . . . . . 119
How Much Sleep Do Children Need? . . . . . . . 120
Establishing a Bedtime Routine . . . . . . . . . . 122
Changing Poor Sleep Habits . . . . . . . . . . . . 123
The Teen Years . . . . . . . . . . . . . . . . . . . 125
Sleepwalking . . . . . . . . . . . . . . . . . . . . . 126
Sleep Terrors . . . . . . . . . . . . . . . . . . . . . 126
Nightmares . . . . . . . . . . . . . . . . . . . . . . 127
Bed-wetting . . . . . . . . . . . . . . . . . . . . . . 128

**12 The Marriage Connection: Supporting Your
Sleepless Spouse** . . . . . . . . . . . . . . . . . . . 131
   Affirm Your Loved One . . . . . . . . . . . . . . . 132
   Examine Your Lifestyle . . . . . . . . . . . . . . . 135
   The Importance of Communication . . . . . . . . 136
   Be Considerate . . . . . . . . . . . . . . . . . . . 137
   Take Action . . . . . . . . . . . . . . . . . . . . . 139
   Be Patient . . . . . . . . . . . . . . . . . . . . . . 140

**13 The Professional Connection: Seeking the Help
You Need** . . . . . . . . . . . . . . . . . . . . . . . 142
   Your Family Physician . . . . . . . . . . . . . . . 142
   Sleep Specialist . . . . . . . . . . . . . . . . . . . 143
   Inside the Sleep Lab . . . . . . . . . . . . . . . . 143
   Procedures and Costs . . . . . . . . . . . . . . . 146
   Conclusion: Bring on the Night! . . . . . . . . . 148

Appendix A: What You Should Know about Medications
and Health Remedies . . . . . . . . . . . . . . . . . . 149

Appendix B: Organizations and Web Sites . . . . . . . . 156

Endnotes . . . . . . . . . . . . . . . . . . . . . . . . . 159
Bibliography . . . . . . . . . . . . . . . . . . . . . . . . 163
Index . . . . . . . . . . . . . . . . . . . . . . . . . . . 166

# Acknowledgments

My heart is filled with gratitude for the assistance of many special people who made the writing and publication of this book a reality.

To my husband, Dick, and my daughters, Taryn and Jill, who prayed for, encouraged, and loved me through the long process of researching and writing this book.

To my incomparable writing group—Margaret Houk, Beth Ziarnik, and Pat Kohls—who put in long hours critiquing the manuscript and contributing thoughtful suggestions in gracious ways.

To my editors at Harold Shaw Publishers, Mary Horner Collins and Bob Bittner, and to Managing Editor Joan Guest, who helped conceive the idea for this book and bring it to completion. I value their professional expertise and their enthusiasm for the possibilities of the published word.

To Dr. Don Derozier, who provided a male perspective to this work and who assisted me with information from his training in psychology and his artful critiquing skill.

To Steven Clark, the registered polysomnographic technologist at Mercy Regional Sleep Disorders Center (Oshkosh, Wisconsin), who invited me behind the scenes to watch a sleep center in action and introduced me to sleep sites on the Internet. And to nighttime technicians Melanie Bloechl and Gary Semb, who allowed me to observe them on the job.

To Dr. Kelli Heindel, who read the manuscript to assure its medical accuracy and readability.

Finally, to my Source of true peace and rest, the Lord Jesus Christ, whose faithful love and abiding presence gives me strength and hope each day *and* night.

# Introduction

Insomnia. It may sneak its way slowly into a person's life, or it may burst in unexpectedly, baggage and all, prepared to stay for a lengthy visit. Either way, it makes for an inconsiderate and unwelcome house-guest.

I know what it is like to lie awake when everyone else in the house is asleep. I understand the feelings of helplessness that fill those lonely hours. In fact, it was my own frustration of living with insomnia that prompted me to learn more about the problem.

I researched the subject thoroughly and interviewed countless insomniacs. I reflected on how my Christian faith fits in and what the Bible has to say about dealing with difficulties. I offer my findings to anyone who battles the same enemy of insomnia as I do.

Insomnia is often called "America's hidden disease." Acccording to the 1998 National Sleep Foundation Omnibus Sleep in America Poll, "two-thirds of American adults reported a sleep-related problem" of varying degrees. That's around 132 million people! The poll also found that 43 percent of that group, or 56 million people, suffer from insomnia specifically.[1] Health authorities say that sleep deprivation may be the number one undiagnosed and untreated medical problem in the country today.

Sleeplessness is now considered the epidemic of our century, reaching crisis proportions. As we near the end of the twentieth century, people now sleep between one and two hours less each night than their ancestors did in the early 1900s. In our twenty-four-hour society, shift work is common and activities once reserved for daylight hours now extend into the dark of night, thanks to the discovery and wide availability of electricity.

Many Americans have deliberately shortened their hours of sleep to have more time for productivity and/or pleasure. As a result, our nation has become sleep-starved. By continually shortchanging ourselves on sleep, we become less alert, slow our reaction time, and reduce our immune system functions, to name only a few negative consequences.

But there's hope for stemming off these unwanted results. Our lifestyles, health, jobs, built-in body clocks, emotional well-being, and environments are factors that make us more or less vulnerable to sleep disturbances. When we become aware of how these issues affect our rest, we can usually improve our sleep quality and its duration. Whether we achieve this on our own or consult a doctor, sleep specialist, or counselor depends on the cause of our sleepless nights. If you need to seek professional help, you will find suggestions for how to find the appropriate expert in chapter 13. If your spouse or child is the sleepless one in your home, I have also included information for assisting them.

You took a positive step toward a better night's sleep when you picked up this book. What you read here will help you start evicting sleeplessness from your life. To do so may involve making some changes in your attitudes, your lifestyle, or your physical condition. But you will face this nighttime intruder armed with solid information, practical direction, and spiritual understanding.

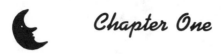 *Chapter One*

# Understanding Your Sleep Connection

From earliest recorded history, human beings have spent about one-third of their lifetimes asleep. This sleep time allows our bodies time to rest from daily physical activity and our minds from mental exercise. During those sleep-filled hours, we become virtually unaware of everything going on around us as we are restored, gathering strength to face the challenges of the next day.

But when our sleep pattern—our "connection" to this time of restoration—is interrupted, real frustration follows. If you're like me and have difficulty getting to sleep or staying asleep, you'll try just about anything to solve the problem. What makes sleep so easy for some and so difficult for others? Why does a certain remedy work for one person but not for another? We want reassurance that we are not alone. We long to welcome the nighttime hours and get a good night's sleep, perhaps for the first time in years.

This book does not seek to offer the last word on insomnia. What it will do, though, is help take away the fear and helplessness that so often accompany sleepless nights. My desire is that by reading these pages you will find both help and hope in your sleepless hours.

## What Is Sleep?

Let's begin by getting a better understanding of the sleep world, that mysterious third part of our daily cycle. By taking time to view the landscape there, we will begin to see possibilities for improving both the *quantity* and *quality* of our sleep.

Imagine your sleep time as the third part of a three-act play. In the first two acts, the stage is bright. It teems with movement and energy as actors enter and exit, play their roles, speak their lines. Then, as the third act begins, the stage darkens. The actors fade until they are barely visible. They no longer move about or interact with one another. This portion of the play seems as endless to those watching it as to those who participate in it. They all welcome the finale, when activity can begin once again.

The term *sleep* means the biological and behavioral state of our bodies when they are at rest, unresponsive to external stimuli. Yet as inactive as sleep may appear, it is far from a static condition. Two distinctly different phases alternate throughout each sleep period. These are called NREM ("non-rapid eye movement") sleep and REM ("rapid eye movement") sleep.

The NREM phase occurs first in the sleep process and progresses through four stages in approximately ninety-minute cycles. These stages, measured by an electroencephalograph (EEG), are distinguished by the size and speed of brain waves produced during sleep. We go to bed where, from a drowsy state, our brain waves begin to slow down, and we slip into stage one. As we sink deeper into sleep, we enter stage two.

# Figure 1: Brain Wave Activity during Sleep

Stage 1 — (NREM sleep) — theta waves

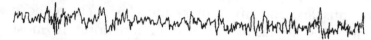

Stage 2 — sleep spindles and K complexes

sleep spindle  K complex

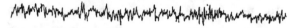

Stage 3 — delta waves
(often combined with stage 4 and called "Delta Sleep")

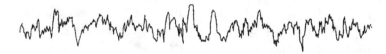

Stage 4 — (REM deep sleep) — random fast waves

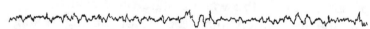

*Source: Mercy Regional Sleep Disorder Center, Oshkosh, Wisconsin, 1997*

The third and fourth stages of NREM sleep are characterized by much larger and slower brain waves, called delta waves. Together these two stages are called "delta sleep" or "deep sleep." During this time, large amounts of growth hormone are secreted, and sleepers require the most stimulation to awaken. Brain activity is minimal, and the body is restored from the effects of its daily activity.

REM sleep begins at the end of stage four, when brain activity increases once more. REM sleep is so-called because the sleeper's eyes move around behind closed eyelids, perhaps following the visual images of dreams. The sleeper's body is almost completely paralyzed during REM sleep except for heart, diaphragm, eye muscles, and involuntary muscles such as those controlling stomach and bladder functions. In most cases, this prevents sleepers from acting out their dreams. (Only in rare instances does movement occur, from sleepwalking to the more serious REM-sleep behavior disorder. For more information on movement disorders, see chapter 5.) During REM sleep, circulation accelerates and body temperature rises. At this stage, the EEG records faster, shallower waves of brain activity. (See Figure 1 on p. 17.)

Although scientists disagree on what exactly dream sleep does for our minds and bodies, they concur that it is important in refreshing us, particularly our brains, to participate in the waking state once again.

In the first ninety-minute cycle of the night, stage four sleep is the longest. After that, each cycle grows shorter in its amount of deep sleep, while stage two and REM sleep increase in duration. As we age, we spend less and less time in deep sleep. Older adults usually sleep more lightly, with little if any deep sleep at all.

# Effects of Too Little Sleep

"I don't consider myself a lonely person," Molly told me, "except in the middle of the night. I wander through my house wishing I could talk to someone. I feel so totally alone and don't know where to turn. Everyone else seems to be blissfully asleep and unaware of my misery. How do they do it?"

Like Molly, those who struggle to sleep often find themselves awake when everyone else in the house is deep in slumber. They spend hour after hour just watching and waiting for the "house lights" to come on—for morning to signal an end to their interminable night hours.

Temporary loss of sleep and its resulting fatigue have a limited effect on our productivity and coping skills, which can be overcome by catching up on just a few hours of sleep. However, when hours of sleeplessness accumulate, each deficiency is exaggerated in exponential proportions. Daytime drowsiness reduces our attention span and impairs our ability to concentrate, react to situations, and solve problems. If fatigue leads to involuntary periods of sleep, however brief, serious consequences may result.

Significant sleep loss interferes with people's jobs and relationships and even threatens their lives. According to the American Sleep Disorders Association, sleep deprivation is responsible for far more vehicle accidents and workplace injuries and deaths than was previously recognized. In fact, people who report chronic insomnia have two-and-a-half times as many automobile accidents as those without sleep problems. A study by the National Highway Traffic Safety Administration found that sleep-deprived people have almost as many accidents as drunk drivers. The U.S.

Department of Transportation estimates that up to 200,000 traffic accidents each year are related to sleep loss. Even more staggering is the fact that 20 percent of all drivers have dozed off at least once behind the wheel.

Major industrial accidents have occurred in the middle of the night as a result of "the human factor," including the tragedy at the Chernobyl nuclear plant in the Ukraine, the Three Mile Island nuclear plant accident, and the *Exxon Valdez*'s grounding on the Alaskan coastline and its resulting massive oil spill. Air-traffic controllers, long-distance truck drivers, shift workers, physicians, and many others often struggle to maintain their ability to work at optimum levels on lower "restorative sleep" levels than their bodies need.

Even though our personalities will not be radically affected by sleep loss—though we may become more short-tempered and impatient—our alertness, reaction time, short-term memory, judgment, and creative thinking skills are impaired to varying extents.

If you suffer from chronic insomnia, this is hardly news to you. You know the internal distress insomnia causes and how it diminishes your quality of life. The question is, What can you do about it? The first step is to find out how much sleep your body requires to function at its best.

## Sleep Deprived?

A recent survey shows that nearly one in three Americans sleeps as little as six hours or less per night during the work week.[1] If we get fewer hours of sleep than our body needs night after night, it can accumulate into a significant "sleep debt." To discover if you are sleep deprived, ask yourself the following questions:

❧ Do I fall asleep within five minutes of going to bed?

❧ Do I feel extremely tired when I should be most alert—before noon and in the early evening?

❧ Do I doze off when I read or watch television?

❧ Do I fall asleep when I ride in a car or when I sit inactively in a public place, like a theater?

❧ Is it more difficult for me to do routine chores than it used to be?

❧ Is it easy for me to sleep in on the weekends, often getting a couple more hours of sleep than I do on weekdays?

❧ Has my mental reaction time slowed down?

❧ Have I experienced memory loss?

If you answered "yes" to three or more of these questions and you sleep a minimum of seven hours each night, you probably have at least a mild sleep disturbance, which is serious enough to warrant medical attention.

## How Much Sleep Do I Need?

Before you can know how much sleep you might be missing out on, you first need to discover how much sleep you actually are getting.

To see how many hours, on average, that you spend sleeping, record the time you go to sleep each night and the time you get up in the morning for one week. At the end of a full week, add up the hours and divide the total by seven. If you function well at your current amount, try cutting back during the next week, either going to bed one hour later or getting up one hour earlier. How do you feel after a shorter night's sleep? after sleeping longer? Experiment to find out how many hours you really need to feel refreshed and operate at your best throughout the day without feeling drowsy.

Don't worry if the amount you need differs from that of others around you. We were created as individuals and, contrary to the "eight-hours-of-sleep rule" we've probably heard all our lives, our bodies vary from one another in their sleep needs. While most people average between seven and eight hours per night, about 5 percent of sleepers function adequately with as few as five hours. A few such "short sleepers" include President Bill Clinton (about five hours per night), lifestyle consultant Martha Stewart (four hours), former British Prime Minister Margaret Thatcher (four hours), and late-night talk-show host Jay Leno (only two to three hours). On the other hand, about 10 percent of the population requires more than nine hours of sleep per night. These are usually creative people who tend to have more dreams at night because of greater time spent in slumber. Most of us fall somewhere in between.

## Sleep Needs Change with Age

Many wonder whether we need different amounts of sleep at different times in our lives. The answer is yes and no. More hours of sleep are needed when our bodies undergo major developmental changes and growth spurts—as infants and adolescents, for example—but the common idea that elderly persons need less sleep than they did when they were younger has proved false.

On the other hand, our *quality* of sleep does change with age. This is at least partially due to some of the medical conditions that arise in older age that interfere with the hours of deepest sleep. Older people tend to awaken earlier and more often, then doze off during the day, setting up a cycle of fragmented sleep that leaves them unrefreshed.

Of course, when we become ill or sustain an injury, we need to give our bodies opportunities for more rest. Stressful periods in our lives also demand that we rest more often than usual.

Whatever our season of life, our goal is to aim for quality as well as quantity of sleep. So, if you're not sleepy, read on to find the help you need to sleep better.

# Chapter Two

# Fixing a Faulty Sleep Connection

Are you tired because you haven't had a good night's sleep for as long as you can remember? Tired because you wander around your house in the middle of the night when everyone else is sound asleep? Tired of being tired?

If you nodded your head wearily in response to these questions, let me offer you an energetic spark of hope. There is something you can do today, right now, to embark on a journey toward achieving several consecutive hours of restorative sleep each night. The first two hopeful steps involve discovering the causes of sleeplessness and what type of insomniac you are. Armed with this information, you will be able to confront your problem, gain the upper hand, and arrest the sleep-robbers.

## Causes of Insomnia

Insomnia's many causes can be grouped under the following categories:

- ✺ Stress (from specific events or a person's life-style)

- ✺ Physical disorders (pain, illness, nervous conditions, breathing problems)

- ✺ Growth and development (puberty, midlife, or menopause)

- ✺ Poor sleep habits (from shift work, nursing, caregiving, jet lag, or working two jobs)

- ✺ Psychological issues (fears, tension, grief, or depression)

- ✺ Environmental issues (drafty room or bad bed that does not sustain healthy sleep)

- ✺ Medications (including certain psychiatric drugs, alcohol, caffeine, and the misuse of sleeping pills)

We will address these subjects individually in the following chapters. For now, our purpose is to learn which causes presently keep you up at night. Knowing the cause determines the direction you should take to find a solution.

## Types of Insomnia

Insomnia can range from an occasional, mildly sleepless night to a long-term, severe condition. Both affect your ability to remain alert during the waking day. Different types of insomnia are defined as transient, short-term, and chronic insomnia. Which best characterizes your pattern of sleeplessness?

*Transient insomnia* lasts for only a few days and is usually the result of acute stress. Abrupt changes in your lifestyle or environment, an illness, jet lag, or the effects of a medication can bring on temporary sleeplessness.

*Short-term insomnia* lingers for one to three weeks at a time. It may return again and is often triggered by more serious losses, such as losing a job, losing a spouse through divorce, or losing a loved one through death. If left unchecked, short-term insomnia may develop into chronic insomnia.

*Chronic insomnia* lasts from three weeks to several years. It is often associated with physical problems such as pain, respiratory trouble, or a sleep disorder. Irregular sleep patterns may trigger chronic insomnia, and it may be a sign of depression. It also may result from the abuse of alcohol, nicotine, caffeine, or other drugs. Effective treatment of insomnia may prevent other problems from getting out of hand. For example, sleep deprivation hinders emotional health, and major depression may be averted if the symptom is managed successfully.

*Difficulty falling asleep* often is a result of a disruptive environment, feeling so "keyed up" that it is hard to unwind, or an irregular sleep schedule. Your sleep patterns can give you clues to what is causing your insomnia.

*If you wake up often throughout the night,* you might look for underlying medical problems, certain sleep disorders or the effects of drugs (even sleep-aid prescriptions) or alcohol. Aging can play a role in frequent waking as well.

*Awakening too early in the morning* usually signals depression, a circadian rhythm disturbance, or regular environmental disruption.

## Charting Your Sleep History

The following questionnaires will help you to further identify the cause and type of your own sleeplessness. Answer the questions as honestly and completely as possible.

────────── **Your Sleep History** ──────────

1. When did your difficulty with sleep begin? Try to remember what was happening in your life at the time.
2. How many nights per week do you have trouble sleeping?
3. Does it occur on certain nights, week after week?
4. What time do you usually go to bed at night? What time do you usually get up in the morning (including weekdays and weekends)?
5. When would you prefer to go to bed and get up if you could set your own sleep schedule?
6. Do you have trouble falling asleep? How long does it usually take?
7. How often do you wake up during the night? Do you have trouble getting back to sleep?
8. Do you often wake up earlier than you want to and find yourself unable to get back to sleep?
9. Do you often feel excessively tired during the day due to lack of sleep?
10. Do you nap during the day? If so, for how long?
11. Is getting too little sleep interfering with your work or social life?
12. Do you have concentration and/or memory problems?
13. Is your mood affected by the amount of sleep you get? Are you irritable, tense, depressed, or confused?
14. Do you do shift work or work nights?

By answering these questions, you have stepped back and observed your sleep patterns objectively. This information is important in your search for better sleep.

The next step involves recording your current sleep habits each day for two weeks.

## Keep a Sleep Journal

Vicky had suffered from sleeplessness for several years, and she invariably looked worn-out. Recently, however, I noticed that her face appeared brighter and she seemed to have more energy.

"Someone suggested that I start keeping a record of my sleep habits," she told me. "It didn't take long before I began to see how certain activities or foods made a difference in how well I slept. I noticed some patterns, made minor changes, and things began to improve. I felt less helpless and more in charge of my ability to sleep."

Sleep research has shown that the most efficient way to find out why people can't sleep is to record sleep practices in a sleep journal (also called a "sleep log" or "sleep diary") for at least two weeks. The information you write in this journal will be a valuable tool in treating your sleeplessness, whether you experiment with self-care or seek help from a professional. (If you are considering a visit to a sleep disorders clinic, you will be asked to record your sleep experiences in a sleep journal prior to arrival.)

Although each night is different, you will probably be surprised by what you learn as you track your day-night cycles of behavior and see their relation to your sleep loss. Simply keeping such a journal helps alleviate any feelings of helplessness you might have regarding your ability to become an effortless sleeper.

You can obtain a printed sleep journal from your physician, or simply create your own based on the information below. Some professionals request that you keep two logs—one for nights, another for days. The questions that follow encompass the entire twenty-four-hour period. Answer them soon after you get up in the morning, recording your general impressions as accurately as possible, guessing when you are unsure.

## Sleep Journal Questions

1. Did you consume any of these substances before you went to bed?
   Caffeine (within 6 hours of bedtime) ___
   Alcohol (within 1 hour of bedtime) ___
   Medication ___ Type _____

2. What time did you go to bed last night?

3. Approximately how many minutes did it take you to fall asleep?

4. How many times did you awaken during the night?

5. What time did you wake up (for the last time) this morning?

6. About how many total hours did you sleep?

7. In general, how did you feel when you woke up: refreshed? somewhat refreshed? unrefreshed?

8. How much time, if any, did you spend napping during the day?

9. Rate your mood and overall functioning during the day on a scale from 1 to 5 (1 = negative/lethargic; 5 = positive/energetic).

## Explore Your Life for Clues

By now you should be convinced that those of us who struggle with insomnia are not alone in our wakefulness. Yet neither do we lie awake at night for exactly the same reasons as anyone else. Just as our individual sleep needs are unique, so the reasons for *not* sleeping vary from person to person.

Sleep specialists act as private investigators to help

us find ways to repay our sleep debt. One of their basic tools is asking questions like the ones that follow. I have adapted various questionnaires and come up with my own versions here to help us begin to investigate on our own. As you examine your lifestyle and physical, emotional, and psychological well-being, you will find more clues to the causes of your sleeplessness.

## Physical Factors

One contributor to sleeplessness is medical or health problems. We may go to the doctor for help with physical problems, yet it's surprising how many people never think to relate these issues to their sleep problems.

──────────── **Medical Problems** ────────────

|  |  | Yes | No |
|---|---|---|---|
| 1. | Do allergy symptoms like congestion, sneezing, or coughing bother you at night? | ☐ | ☐ |
| 2. | Does arthritis, joint, or back pain keep you awake? | ☐ | ☐ |
| 3. | Does frequent acid indigestion, reflux, or nausea disturb your sleep? | ☐ | ☐ |
| 4. | Are your legs restless at bedtime? | ☐ | ☐ |
| 5. | Do you awaken yourself or your spouse by kicking your legs during the night? | ☐ | ☐ |
| 6. | Is your bedding messed up when you wake up in the morning? | ☐ | ☐ |
| 7. | Are you a heavy snorer? Has your spouse noticed that you stop breathing in the night? | ☐ | ☐ |
| 8. | Do you experience repetitive nightmares? | ☐ | ☐ |
| 9. | Do you grind or clench your teeth at night? | ☐ | ☐ |

|  | Yes | No |
|---|---|---|
| 10. Have you walked in your sleep as an adult? | ☐ | ☐ |
| 11. Do you have a particular medical problem that keeps you awake at night? | ☐ | ☐ |
| 12. Do you take medications that contain caffeine, ephedrine, or amphetamine? | ☐ | ☐ |

If you answered yes to any of these questions, you have a clue to a possible physical cause for your sleepless nights. Make an appointment for a complete physical if you have not had one in the past year, and be sure to mention your sleep difficulties.

The amount of information about insomnia available today far surpasses that of just a few years ago, and your general physician can give you help or refer you to a sleep specialist, if necessary. To further explore this aspect of insomnia, turn to chapters 4 and 5 for further discussion of medical causes and various sleep disorders.

Closely related to the medical causes of insomnia are the effects of sleep medications on how well we sleep. Consider these questions about sleep aids:

- ❧ How often do you use a prescription sleep medication?

- ❧ How often do you use an over-the-counter sleeping pill?

- ❧ How often do you use alcohol as a sleep aid?

You may be surprised to discover the positive or negative impact of medications by reading the information in appendix A, by studying package inserts, and by discussing sleep aids you currently use with your doctor or pharmacist.

## Emotional Issues

Psychological factors play a large role in how well we cope with stress, which is the leading cause of insomnia today. If depression and anxiety are contributing to your sleep loss, your insomnia may well be solved by getting treatment for its underlying psychological causes. I was comforted to learn that just because we can't sleep due to psychological problems does not mean we are crazy or psychotic.[1] Use the following questions to understand better your emotional well-being.

———————— **Depression** ————————

|  | T | F |
|---|---|---|
| 1. I am often sad and can't snap out of it. | ☐ | ☐ |
| 2. I am pessimistic about the future. | ☐ | ☐ |
| 3. I feel disappointed in myself. | ☐ | ☐ |
| 4. I believe that others are disappointed in me. | ☐ | ☐ |
| 5. I am dissatisfied or bored most of the time. | ☐ | ☐ |
| 6. I often feel bad or unworthy and blame myself when things go wrong. | ☐ | ☐ |
| 7. Sometimes I think about harming myself. | ☐ | ☐ |
| 8. I cry a lot. | ☐ | ☐ |
| 9. I get irritated more easily than I used to. | ☐ | ☐ |
| 10. I have lost interest in other people. | ☐ | ☐ |
| 11. I have more difficulty making decisions than I used to. | ☐ | ☐ |
| 12. I've stopped taking care of myself. | ☐ | ☐ |
| 13. My feelings are affecting my work and relationships. | ☐ | ☐ |
| 14. I wake up one or more hours earlier than usual and can't get back to sleep. | ☐ | ☐ |
| 15. I feel tired even when there is no reason to be. | ☐ | ☐ |

|   |   | T | F |
|---|---|---|---|
| 16. | My appetite is poor (or, I eat excessively). | ☐ | ☐ |
| 17. | I've lost interest in sex. | ☐ | ☐ |
| 18. | I feel worse in the morning, better in the evening. | ☐ | ☐ |
| 19. | I have trouble getting things done that used to be easy for me. | ☐ | ☐ |
| 20. | One or more of my close relatives has been treated for depression. | ☐ | ☐ |

## Anxiety

|   |   | T | F |
|---|---|---|---|
| 1. | I often feel upset or tense without knowing why. | ☐ | ☐ |
| 2. | Sometimes my heart races uncontrollably. | ☐ | ☐ |
| 3. | My hands are often sweaty, clammy, or extremely cold. | ☐ | ☐ |
| 4. | I often have a lump in my throat. | ☐ | ☐ |
| 5. | I have difficulty slowing down and relaxing. | ☐ | ☐ |
| 6. | I often feel insecure or anxious. | ☐ | ☐ |
| 7. | I often feel ill at ease. | ☐ | ☐ |
| 8. | I worry about things I've said that might have hurt somebody's feelings. | ☐ | ☐ |
| 9. | I often feel tired without any reason. | ☐ | ☐ |
| 10. | I tend to worry, even over things I realize don't matter. | ☐ | ☐ |
| 11. | I worry about a possible misfortune. I'm apprehensive about the future. | ☐ | ☐ |

Make an appointment with a professional counselor if several of the statements in the surveys above seem true for you. Sometimes just talking things over and learning to deal with life's challenges helps overcome sleeplessness. Other times an antidepressant will improve your sleep almost immediately. (That doesn't mean you will have to rely on such medication for the rest of your life.)

Take advantage of free depression screening when it is offered by area medical centers. Using questionnaires, educational presentations, and brief personal consultations, they will be able to refer you to resources available in your community. Chapter 9 looks further into the psychological and emotional causes of insomnia.

## Balanced Lifestyle

Lifestyle issues rank high on the list of reasons we can't sleep at night. When we review our schedules, we realize that sometimes we don't keep our times of work, play, and rest in balance. When stress is allowed to increase without release, it can keep us awake. Like breathing, our lives should not be all "inhale"; we also need to "exhale" regularly. We need a "breather" at the end of each day, each week, each year. Our bodies were not created to go full speed without rest.

──────────────── **Lifestyle Survey** ────────────────

|  | T | F |
|---|---|---|
| 1. I feel I'm under a great deal of stress at work (trouble with the boss, long hours, etc.) or at home (marital arguments, demands from kids, money worries, etc.). | ☐ | ☐ |
| 2. I smoke (number of)____ cigarettes per day. I began smoking ____ years ago. | ☐ | ☐ |
| 3. I consume coffee, tea, cola, or other caffeinated drinks or foods in the afternoon and/or evening. | ☐ | ☐ |

|  | T | F |
|---|---|---|
| 4. On average, I drink more than two cocktails, beers, or glasses of wine per day. | ☐ | ☐ |
| 5. I exercise vigorously less than twice a week. | ☐ | ☐ |
| 6. I often work more than ten hours a day or more than six days a week. | ☐ | ☐ |
| 7. I'm generally serious; I rarely do anything just for fun. | ☐ | ☐ |
| 8. I take fewer than two weeks of vacation a year. | ☐ | ☐ |
| 9. I'm struggling with some relationships with my family, friends, or coworkers. | ☐ | ☐ |

If several of these statements are true for you, stop and reflect. Our bodies perform best—at work *and* rest—if we are mindful about what we put into them. Substances like alcohol, caffeine, and nicotine lessen our "sleepability," while exercise, relaxation, and doing things for others promote rest. (Did you know that the energy spent in helping others often relieves stress that may contribute to sleeplessness?) Check out chapter 6 for some more practical ways to adjust your lifestyle for a good night's sleep.

Another related lifestyle issue is sleep hygiene. Do you dread going to bed? Terrorized that you won't sleep? Our *sleep hygiene* refers primarily to how conducive our personal habits, thoughts, and environment are to our sleep. How we approach bedtime can make a big difference in our sleep success. Positive attitudes toward the sleep process are crucial, yet they are often overlooked. Some of us grow conditioned to dreading bedtime, rather than welcoming it. In the next chapter, we'll look at how we can change our minds about insomnia and overcome the fears.

You stand on the edge of finally getting some much-desired, much-needed sleep. By answering the questions in this chapter and starting your sleep journal, you are on your way to finding rest.

# Chapter Three

# The Mental Connection

*Changing Your Attitudes
about Sleeplessness*

For those of us who are sleep-challenged, the possibility that we may not get a good night's sleep lurks in the back of our minds even during daylight hours. It crouches at our bedside, daring us to climb under the covers. We fear it. We fight it. We try to forget about it, but it is always there.

What can we do to rid ourselves of this invisible enemy? Incredibly, sometimes just changing our minds about this "monster" can free us from its power.

As I studied insomnia, my efforts to gain information changed my outlook in ways I didn't foresee. I was able to identify and then correct some faulty ways of thinking. When combined with faith—an element I'll discuss in chapter 10—this insight became an effective weapon in my fight for sleep.

Our attitudes toward sleep develop over many years, fashioned by our experiences, our personalities, and any information on the subject—correct or not—that we have recorded in our brains. These attitudes affect our ability to cope with the every-night occurrence of bedtime. Whether we greet it with a welcome embrace or push it away in dread often depends on our expectations about how we will sleep and whether we will awake the next morning refreshed.

Because our thoughts are powerful forces in getting a good night's sleep, we need to make sure they are accurate. In this chapter we will examine some common problem areas and suggest positive alternatives and solutions.

## You're Not Alone

When you wander through your house in the middle of the night, staring out on the dark silhouettes of homes in your neighborhood, you might feel as if you are the only person awake for miles around, that you are a bit abnormal. *Everyone else is sound asleep. What's wrong with me?* you think.

I used to feel that way. Then I learned that two-thirds of the adult population of the United States struggles with sleeplessness to some degree, and half of all Americans suffer insomnia at one time or another.[1] We have plenty of company in our lonely nights. We aren't an exception to the rest of the human race. In fact, our problems aren't strange or at all unusual. And they are nothing new.

For centuries people have struggled to get enough sleep. I realized this when I took a closer look at many of the sleepless nights recorded in the Bible. Thousands of years ago, Job—a man remembered today for the extreme suffering he endured—spoke these words from the depths of physical, emotional, and spiritual anguish: "When I lie down I think, 'How long before I get up?' The night drags on, and I toss till dawn" (Job 7:4). Or consider this sigh of discouragement from the book of Psalms: "I am worn out from groaning; all night long I flood my bed with weeping" (Psalm 6:6). According to the Bible, even ancient kings (Xerxes and Darius, in particular) had sleepless nights.

I find comfort in the company of these ancient insomniacs. And when I discovered that many researchers today are investigating sleep problems and making significant progress toward solving them, I found hope in their "company" as well. Foundations, associations, councils, and clinics exist to fight our battle with us. Sleep science is multidisciplinary, involving physicians of various specialties (pulmonary and psychiatric, to name two). Also, corporations—from mattress manufacturers to pharmaceutical companies—continually create new products to improve people's sleep based on the latest research. The sleep problem-solving industry is far larger than I had anticipated. That is reassuring. Perhaps it will find a cure.

## Don't Try So Hard

Ironically, the more we try to capture a few hours of sleep, the more elusive it becomes. Every expert I have talked to and every resource I've read agree on this important advice: If you want to sleep, stop thinking about it. Stop trying so hard. Instead, focus your mind on other things.

"Oh, sure," Jenny replied when her doctor offered her this advice. "The more I try to think about something else, the more I can't think about anything *but* getting some sleep!"

Can you relate to Jenny? Many of us can. The longer we try unsuccessfully to avoid thinking about it, the greater frustration we experience. Turmoil takes over our thought processes. We lose self-confidence and hope. We grow depressed, irritable, and even angry in the face of our apparent helplessness.

Yet just as figure skaters train their bodies to trace complicated and precise figures on ice, so we have the ability to train our minds to allow sleep to come. Cognitive therapists have found thought modification to be particularly helpful for those whose sleep difficulties arise from erroneous attitudes and thought patterns.

So how *do* you stop trying to sleep? One solution is to aim your attention in another direction. Allow yourself to be distracted by something else by trying the following:

- ❧ Read for awhile, choosing your reading material wisely—nothing too stimulating.

- ❧ Count or make lists. In your mind, print large numbers or letters on a chalkboard in a monotonous rhythm.

- ❧ Listen to soft music. There are countless recordings made just to relax listeners to sleep.

- ❧ Let your thoughts drift aimlessly without allowing them to settle on any one thing.

- ❧ If a thought takes hold and won't let go, jot it down so you can reflect on it in the light of the next day. If a specific concern troubles you, try praying about the matter and leaving it in God's hands.

- ❧ Picture yourself in a calm setting, such as a seashore or a forest, and listen for the quiet, soothing sounds around you.

- ❧ Breathe deeply and slowly for several minutes.

## Avoid "Fear of Insomnia"

The fear of losing sleep, *agrypniaphobia,* can thwart our best attempts to catch some Zzzs. Fear evokes a fight-or-flight response and increases our supply of adrenaline, thus decreasing our ability to rest.

But here is an antidote to that fear. Even if you don't sleep at all for one night, you *will* be able to get through the next day. Researchers have proved this in laboratory studies where they kept volunteers awake through the night and then measured the subjects' abilities to perform certain tasks the next day.

I discovered this firsthand when my children were very young and my husband went out of town on business. After I spent a night unable to sleep, I worried anxiously about the day ahead. Yet I found myself able to keep up with my children (one an active toddler) and perform my other responsibilities as well. Since that time I no longer panic if I am sleepless for a whole night. (The exception is, of course, if you are mounting up a significant sleep debt. Eventually your abilities *will* begin to deteriorate.)

How do you react if you don't sleep well one night? Do you begin to panic? "How can I function if I don't get my eight hours of shut-eye? I've just *got* to get some sleep tonight, but what if I don't? How will I get through tomorrow? I'm scared to crawl into bed, afraid the same thing will happen again." Such thoughts are often prophetic: the more you fret, the less you sleep. This can lead to a vicious cycle of expecting not to sleep, growing more tense, temporarily experiencing insomnia, then developing long-term insomnia as a result.

If you haven't been able to sleep for a few weeks

or longer, you may have learned some negative patterns without being aware of it. Has your bed become for you a place of failure and frustration because of your inability to sleep? This is what experts call "conditioned insomnia." You have programmed yourself to become wakeful as you approach bedtime. To see if this is true of you, think about where you sleep best. Is it in your own bed or somewhere else? If you drift off better away from home or even in your living room recliner, you may be experiencing conditioned insomnia.

At Northwestern University, Dr. Richard Bootzin developed an effective treatment for conditioned insomnia, based on stimulus-control therapy. Dr. Bootzin advised his patients to go to bed only when sleepy and to use their beds only for sleeping (not reading, watching TV, or eating). If they couldn't sleep, they were to get up, move to another room, and stay up until they were really sleepy, then return to bed. If sleep still didn't come, they were to get out of bed again and repeat this procedure as often as necessary throughout the night. In this way they would learn to associate their beds with falling asleep easily and quickly rather than with frustration and sleeplessness.

In addition, Bootzin's patients were told to set the alarm and get up at the same time every morning, regardless of how much or how little they slept during the night, thereby helping their bodies to maintain a constant sleep-wake rhythm. They also were cautioned not to nap during the day.

Studies of patients using the Bootzin technique reveal that they showed marked improvement in their ability to sleep within about two weeks.[2]

## Correct Your Misperceptions

Although you may have been taught that you must get eight hours of sleep each night to feel refreshed and be fully functional throughout the next day, remember that sleep needs vary from person to person. You may be perfectly able to get by on less.

Do you believe your health and well-being depend on a good night's sleep? Some of your belief may be justified. However, this can be a self-defeating approach to your situation. Think about why you feel this way. Is your expectation realistic? Watch that you don't blame everything that goes wrong in your life on not getting enough sleep.

We have a tendency to magnify our problems when we haven't slept well. We enlarge them out of proportion. Studies have found that, though insomnia impairs concentration, memory, judgment, and mood, actual performance does not necessarily deteriorate. This holds true even when our perception suggests otherwise. Experiment with this by putting aside your concern about your lack of sleep and, later, evaluating how you handled the responsibilities of your day.

You may find it helpful to write out your current thoughts about sleep and its role in your life. Describe your feelings about not getting enough sleep for one or two nights or more. Whenever you are able, test each perception to see if it is indeed valid. As you file correct information in your brain, you will begin to gain a sense of control over and greater tolerance for your sleeplessness.

## Putting Your Brain to Bed

When it comes to winding down to sleep, our mind

is often the culprit that won't let us relax. It keeps going, worrying, pondering, creating all sorts of restlessness. To prevent this, examine your current bedtime habits and begin to make some adjustments where necessary.

Whether we realize it or not, we all perform bedtime rituals. We brush our teeth, wash our faces, change into our nightclothes, and then climb into bed. But what happens when these habits trigger sleeplessness? What happens if, as soon as we begin preparing for bed, we are already worrying about whether or not we will get to sleep? With our hearts and minds racing, the experience becomes a self-fulfilling prophecy, and we *don't* sleep. The pattern repeats itself the next night, and we end up feeling like failures. How often I've thought, "Even babies can sleep! What's my problem?"

Think about it. We establish bedtime rituals for our children. We give them baths, help them brush their teeth, say their prayers with them, read them a bedtime story, then kiss them goodnight. Some children are nodding off before the light goes out.

Why not make this a goal for yourself? Examine your own bedtime habits. Which do you consider essential? Might one or more be likely to cause more wakefulness than relaxation? Now is the time to make some adjustments. If your nightly cup of tea contains caffeine, try changing to an herbal or decaffeinated tea. If you find yourself waking in the night to use the bathroom and then have trouble falling asleep again, try eliminating all beverages for a few hours before bedtime. Whatever you do in the evening should be aimed at relaxation. For more ideas on bedtime preparation, see chapter 6.

## Don't Play the Victim

When we suffer from a problem for a period of time, we often use the role of "helpless victim" as a coping mechanism. Do you ever ask others to excuse your short temper because you didn't get enough sleep? Do you deny responsibility for your actions because you didn't sleep well? These are signals that you may be unconsciously using your sleeplessness to your own advantage.

Believe it or not, there are those among us, says Dr. Julius Segal, a sleep expert at the National Institute of Mental Health, for whom sleeplessness has become a status symbol. These people think that if we take life seriously, as we are "supposed to," we will naturally suffer from insomnia. It's a sign of success, like an ulcer or a coronary.

Other people subconsciously take pride in their insomnia, believing it reflects the importance of their career, the significance of their lifestyle, or their uniqueness as an individual. They may bask in the sympathy their affliction generates in those around them.

## Attitude Adjustment

Discovering what we think about our inability to sleep may not be a pleasant task, but the process is an important key to healing.

Investigate your own attitudes toward your insomnia. Perhaps your thought patterns need readjustment. Write out your feelings, fears, and frustrations, your hopes and dreams. By identifying your own counterproductive thoughts, you take your first step toward recovering a positive attitude about sleep.

Envision how you might behave if you were well rested. Think about what you have learned. Then join me as we consider the next step: the physical connection.

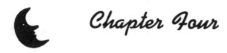 *Chapter Four*

# The Physical Connection, Part 1

## *Checking for Medical Causes*

"The beginning of health is sleep," an old Irish proverb says. How true! When we don't get enough sleep, our bodies show signs of wear. Fatigue causes us to become increasingly vulnerable to illness and life-endangering accidents. Yet sometimes our bodies themselves hold the reasons for our inadequate rest. To find out if that is the case, it's important to explore the physical dimension of our sleeplessness.

Many people hesitate to go to their doctors with such an "insignificant" complaint as being unable to sleep. Perhaps they're embarrassed to admit to such a problem. But Thomas Roth, director of the Sleep Disorders Research Center at Henry Ford Hospital in Detroit warns, "People have no idea how important sleep is to their lives. . . . Good health demands good sleep. Conversely, lack of sleep has serious, often life-threatening consequences."[1]

So the doctor's office is a good place to start a search for a good night's sleep. Physicians are becoming more proficient in finding the reasons behind their patients' specific sleep problems and directing them toward appropriate treatment.

In this chapter we will examine some physical factors that affect the quality of our slumber—gender, age, pain, illness, allergies, and asthma.

## Gender Differences

"Men are from Mars, women are from Venus," John Gray declares in his best-selling book of the same title. Indeed, men and women were created as compatible creatures who differ greatly in their makeup. It makes sense, then, that their sleep troubles will differ also.

While sleep patterns vary from individual to individual, women tend to mention their episodes of insomnia more often than men. However, studies have shown that males generally have worse sleep habits than females, at least until about age sixty-five. After that, the contrast between the two genders lessens. (One reason men register fewer incidences of insomnia than women may be that the American culture discourages men from discussing health problems that make them appear vulnerable or weak.)

When it comes to breathing as a cause of sleep difficulties, women come out ahead of men. The hormone progesterone is thought to play a significant role in protecting females from respiratory difficulties while they sleep. Throughout their lives, females have fewer sleep-related breathing disorders than males, and fewer female babies are victims of sudden infant death syndrome (SIDS) than their male counterparts.

Until menopause, hormone fluctuations play a role in how well women sleep. The hormonal imbalance that occurs during the menstrual cycle can cause sleep deprivation, according to Sharon Schutte of Thomas

Jefferson University's Sleep Disorders Center, and women who suffer from premenstrual syndrome (PMS) are more likely to experience a poorer quality and lesser amount of sleep in the days preceding menstruation.

Pregnancy presents its own unique challenges. During the first trimester, most expectant mothers experience increased daytime drowsiness. During the second trimester, they require more sleep at night, probably because of the energy demands of the new life growing within them. In the last trimester, the baby's increased activity and the mother's anatomical changes may interfere with sleeping positions and begin to cause breathing disruptions.

My own sleep struggles started during my first pregnancy. Like many expectant women, I had difficulty finding a comfortable position for my changing body shape. As my baby grew and pressed against my bladder, I had to visit the bathroom more often in the night. Then my daughter arrived and awakened me at irregular intervals each night for several weeks. These episodes confused my sleep-wake rhythm. Indeed, experts have observed that pregnancy often initiates sleep disruptions that become chronic if not corrected early on.

Later, as women enter middle age, they encounter a host of new sleep challenges. During menopause, and even in the years preceding its onset, hormonal changes often trigger various sleep disturbances, from night sweats (the nocturnal version of hot flashes) to a generally higher anxiety level. Though hormone replacement therapy is effective in resolving many menopausal symptoms, such as hot flashes, HRT does not resolve every sleep difficulty.

Following menopause, women are more at risk of

having sleep apnea than earlier in their lives. Men are more prone to developing sleep apnea, REM-sleep behavior disorder, and periodic limb movements, all of which interfere with sleep quality without the sleeper necessarily being aware of it.

## Sleep Patterns and Older Adults

"I've always been a light sleeper," a friend in her mid-sixties told me. "But now I seem to be awake in the night more than I'm asleep."

Almost everyone notices a change in their sleep patterns as they grow older. Is it true that we need less sleep as we get older? While the *need* for sleep does not change as people age, the *quality* of sleep diminishes, leaving us feeling less refreshed as we grow older. As early as their fifties, people begin waking more often at night and dozing off more readily in the daytime. Dr. Peter Hauri, director of Mayo Clinic's Insomnia Research and Treatment Program, has stated that some older adults have little awakenings dozens of times in the night, lasting fifteen seconds or less. This may give them the impression of having been awake all night when in reality they have gotten a good amount of sleep.

Unfortunately, many older adults build up a significant "sleep debt" as they experience less of the deep, dreamless sleep. Deep sleep is the time when the body is restored, the skin repaired, and bone and muscle built. Endocrinologist Eve Van Cauter calls deep sleep "the ultimate antiaging therapy."[2] Without enough of it, the body is more vulnerable to many of the debilitating diseases of old age.

Many factors contribute to less and poorer sleep as people mature. Older adults' nightly drop in body temperature often becomes less distinct, perhaps as the result of a more sedentary lifestyle. A lack of exercise also prevents their bodies from tiring physically, which inhibits their ability to sleep soundly.

A recent study by Stanford University's School of Medicine found that sedentary older adults who walked or did aerobics four times a week on a prescribed program improved their sleep after sixteen weeks. Those who participated slept about an hour longer each night and cut their sleep onset time in half.

Maintaining a regular schedule of sleeping and waking is more difficult in the retirement years, but it is just as important as it was before. Sleeping in to make up for lost sleep the night before or taking more than one nap a day can significantly impair one's sleep-wake rhythm and contribute to chronic insomnia.

Insomnia is not a necessary part of the aging process. If you or a loved one is experiencing sleeplessness, a professional evaluation can be an invaluable first step in helping you get sufficient rest.

## Pain, Illness, and Insomnia

Arthritis, back pain, a headache, an intestinal virus, or even the common cold can cause our daily activities to suffer significantly. Naturally, they may well disturb our sleep as well.

Any type of pain—acute or chronic—can interfere with our ability to fall asleep and remain asleep. Pain often only allows us to drift in and out of a state of drowsy wakefulness, preventing us from sinking into a deep sleep. After such little rest, we feel pain more acutely, perhaps because our bodies are less able to cope with it then. They haven't had the chance to recharge and renew themselves.

Aspirin, ibuprofen, acetaminophen, or a physician-prescribed pain reliever are frequently used for this discomfort. However, sometimes pain can be cured without pharmaceutical intervention. For example, certain headaches can be "headed off" by sleeping on your back or using a pillow that is indented in the center, designed to relieve neck strain. Your physician might recommend special exercises to reduce pressure and thereby decrease pain.

Illness can also interfere with sleep patterns. If our immune system is to function at its optimum level, we must get a minimum amount of sleep. When we are ill, our bodies need even more rest to hasten the healing process. Yet many medical conditions make sleep more elusive. The discomfort of illnesses—from severe heartburn to bronchitis to a urinary tract infection—can cause persistent or frequent episodes of wakefulness. Treating such conditions sets the stage for sleep to return. If our insomnia began with the onset of a medical problem, attending to it could mean relief from our sleepless nights.

Living with chronic pain or illness is enough of a physical, social, and psychological challenge without the added burden of insomnia. If you have difficulty coping, try to find a pain treatment protocol that will enable a good night's rest.

My friend Pam has suffered with chronic back pain for many years, intense enough that it kept her from falling asleep at night. "I found I couldn't go to sleep if I had even a small amount of pain," she told me. "I used to wait until I couldn't take the pain any longer, then I would get up and take something. When I finally got to sleep, I would wake up four hours later when the pain medication wore off. I began by taking aspirin. When that didn't work any longer, I switched to acetaminophen, then to acetaminophen with codeine or to muscle relaxers. With the help of my doctor, I learned to identify each kind of pain I was feeling, whether it was muscle pain or something else. Now I can treat it more effectively."

Other people with chronic pain have found help by joining a support group, keeping a journal, learning to maintain a positive attitude, developing their sense of humor, receiving counseling, or undergoing massage therapy. As you grow better able to conquer, modify, or accept your disability, you will find yourself better able to cope and to obtain sufficient rest.

## Power in Weakness

As a Christian, I believe that God is able to heal people of pain and disease. Certainly many people bear witness to miraculous cures. When Jesus walked on this earth two thousand years ago, he healed many people who crossed his path. Some were healed by the touch of his hand, others by a word he spoke. Yet others remained sick or disabled. Even the apostle Paul—the writer of many New Testament books of the Bible—endured what he called a "thorn in the flesh," which some think was a physical infirmity. He pleaded three times for God to remove it from him, but God said no, adding that "My grace is sufficient for you, for my power is made perfect in weakness" (2 Corinthians 12:9).

So it is today. One person's prayer is answered, and another's is not. Although we can't discern the why— "Why was her pain healed and not my own?"—we can learn to rest in hope and peace, as Paul did: "For Christ's sake, I delight in weaknesses. . . . For when I am weak, then I am strong" (v. 10).

I'm not suggesting that those who struggle with infirmity should deny or suppress feelings of frustration, even anger. I believe God welcomes our honest emotions, and he listens to our fervent, faith-filled prayers, even when our faith is as tiny as a mustard seed. The health of our *faith* almost always seems to be Jesus' primary concern. And faith can be expressed in persistent prayer for healing, even while it is willing to accept the present reality of suffering. Those who seek God will find that he grants hope for change—in body, in heart, and in our capacity to find physical and spiritual rest.

## Allergies

Breathing difficulties from allergies often become more bothersome at night and can significantly disrupt sleep unless effective treatment is sought.

Whether you suffer from seasonal or year-round allergies, the time and money spent on learning what triggers your reactions will be well spent. I have done so with good success. You may have to experiment with different treatments to bring your symptoms under control.

Specialists' number one suggestion for overcoming allergy symptoms is to avoid those irritants that set in motion the stuffy nose, congestion, sneezing, or itching—whatever keeps you awake at night. This usually also involves one or more of the following:

- Investing in a clean-air machine and/or air conditioning.
- Covering your mattress and box springs with plastic to prevent dust mites and mold build-up.

❧ Finding an antihistamine that suppresses your symptoms to a manageable level. (An added advantage for people who struggle with sleep is that many antihistamines have a sedating effect.)

❧ Undergoing desensitizing shots (also known as *immunotherapy*).

## Asthma

Asthmatics' breathing difficulties often come from environmental allergens and irritants (for example, dust mites, mold, mildew, pet dander, or cold air), postnasal drip from sinusitis, or the reflux of stomach contents into the airways, among others. Because asthmatics' airways are sensitive to irritation, when these airways become inflamed, they produce excess mucus and impair breathing.

Asthma researcher Richard J. Martin, M.D., of the National Jewish Center for Immunology and Respiratory Medicine, says that about 75 percent of asthmatics have breathing problems at least one night a week; 40 percent suffer every night.[3]

The body's internal clock also seems to play a role in nocturnal asthma problems. While normal lung function drops about 8 percent during sleep, asthmatic lung function may be cut by half, causing serious consequences. Also, the natural hormones that reduce inflammation and help keep airways open (epinephrine and cortisol, for example) reach their lowest levels in the middle of the night. Hormones that narrow the airways and generate mucus production (like histamine) increase at night.[4]

What can you do if your asthma symptoms worsen at night?

- ❧ Inform your physician or asthma specialist.

- ❧ Try using an inhaler prior to bedtime and as symptoms occur.

- ❧ Because asthmatics are also allergy prone, follow the suggestions for allergy sufferers listed above.

- ❧ Ask your doctor about oral medications that effectively treat nighttime asthma.

- ❧ Treat any underlying conditions such as sinusitis, sleep apnea, and stomach reflux, which trigger breathing difficulties.

Be aware that some common asthma medications list sleeplessness as a side-effect. If you have this reaction, your physician may change your dosage, substitute a different prescription, or reschedule when you take your medication.

Becoming aware of medical problems we may have is one part of getting more rest. Beyond the factors mentioned in this chapter, other problems often exist in people's bodies that cause them to lose sleep. These maladies are recognized in the growing field of sleep science as "sleep disorders." Read on to find out more about specific manifestations and treatments of these physical challenges.

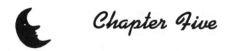

# Chapter Five

# The Physical Connection, Part 2

*Understanding Sleep Disorders*

Even when we insomniacs manage to fall asleep, any one of a number of nocturnal ailments—at least eighty-four, in fact—may interrupt our slumber. These are collectively referred to as "sleep disorders." We'll look at nine of them here, along with their symptoms and suggested treatments. (For a detailed discussion, consult a reference known as *The International Classification of Sleep Disorders.*)

## Sleep Apnea

Meg was awakened night after night by her husband's loud snoring. She began noticing that Rob often seemed to stop breathing, would sometimes gasp for air, then resume his snoring. She mentioned this pattern of sleep behavior to her doctor, who suggested that they make an appointment with a sleep specialist. Rob discovered that he had sleep apnea, one of the most serious and prevalent of sleep disorders.

One person in twelve has some form of sleep apnea, a condition in which the airway in the throat briefly but repeatedly collapses during sleep. The term *apnea* refers to the cessation of respiration; the sleeper actually stops breathing for several seconds at a time. These episodes may last from ten seconds to a couple minutes at one time. Some sufferers do not breathe for three-quarters of their sleep time.[1]

These brief awakenings may occur hundreds of times a night, yet people don't usually remember them. Rather, they complain about excessive daytime drowsiness and may, in fact, fall asleep off and on throughout the day. It is very common for sleepers to be made aware of their apnea symptoms by their co-sleepers.

Poor muscle tension, which allows the throat to collapse during sleep and cut off the air intake, is a primary cause of obstructive sleep apnea. This could result from obesity or anatomical problems, such as a large uvula (the tissue that hangs from the soft palate in the back of the throat), a tongue set too far back in the mouth so it is sucked in when the person breathes, narrow airways, or fat deposits along the airway. Dr. Rafael Pelayo of the Stanford Sleep Clinic says it is unclear whether apnea is caused by obesity alone or in combination with oversized throat tissues, a thick neck, or jaw structure.[2]

Sleep apnea is serious because of its relation to heart disease. Blood pressure rises significantly during each apnea episode due to the lack of oxygen in the bloodstream. This strains the heart, which could lead to a heart attack. Patients with sleep apnea have three times as many traffic accidents as the rest of the population, according to researchers at the University of Wisconsin. And people with undiagnosed sleep apnea are seven times more likely to have multiple accidents, says Terry Young, the professor who authored the study. Only 10 to 15 percent of people with the disorder have been diagnosed, Young notes.[3]

People of any age may suffer from sleep apnea, but the chance of its occurring increases sharply with age. Before women go through menopause, male sufferers of sleep apnea outnumber them about thirty to one. However, after menopause, the gap between them narrows, as women experience increased episodes of apnea.

## Symptoms of Sleep Apnea

There are some typical symptoms that are linked to sleep apnea. See if any of these sound familiar to you.

- Extremely loud snoring interrupted by pauses in breathing, then gasps
- Excessive daytime sleepiness
- Complaints of insomnia, waking up often but not knowing why
- Morning headaches
- Absence of dreams
- High blood pressure
- Irritability and/or depression
- Difficulty remembering things and/or concentrating
- Impotence and/or loss of sex drive
- Falling asleep while driving

If you or your doctor think you may have sleep apnea, the best way to diagnose it is for you to spend a night in a sleep lab. A polysomnography exam will record your brain waves, the number of times you stop breathing, your blood oxygen levels, heart rate, and temperature, among other things. From this information, a sleep specialist can prescribe a regimen to treat your condition, if warranted.

Some cases of sleep apnea may be resolved by losing weight or learning to sleep on your side. More severe cases may require wearing a dental appliance to bring your lower jaw forward and keep your tongue from falling back into your throat. Many apneacs are fitted with a mask that delivers pressurized air to their lungs, keeping their airways open. This device, called "continuous positive air pressure" (CPAP), effectively treats most cases of sleep apnea.

Surgery may be used as a last resort. One type widens the airway by reducing the size of the uvula, soft palate, or both. However, this is effective only about 50 percent of the time. A newer procedure involves getting rid of excess tissue with a laser. It is an office procedure, less painful and less expensive than the first kind, but not necessarily an effective way to cure moderate to severe sleep apnea. The most serious cases of obstructive sleep apnea, where heart failure and extremely high blood pressure are symptomatic, may require a tracheostomy.

In each case, you should undergo a post-surgery sleep study to determine its success in treating your apnea.

Central sleep apnea differs from obstructive sleep apnea discussed above. The airway remains open, but the muscles in the diaphragm and chest stop working. As the level of oxygen in the blood falls, the brain signals the sleeper to awaken and begin breathing again. Central sleep apnea is more common in older people, affecting almost one-fourth of the population over sixty years of age. For most, the problem is mild, but it becomes more frequent and severe in those with other medical and neurological disorders.[4]

Researchers now believe there may be a link between sleep apnea and sudden infant death syndrome (SIDS). A study conducted by Dr. Susan Redline of Case Western Reserve University found that every child who suffered from SIDS or another nighttime breathing problem had at least one relative with sleep apnea, although not every baby whose relative has sleep apnea is at risk for SIDS. The American Academy of Pediatrics recommends that all healthy infants be positioned on their sides or backs for sleep.[5]

Children may suffer from apnea as well. Their symptoms include labored breathing, pauses in breathing while they sleep, or extreme sleepiness during the day. Such children sometimes are presumed lazy or "slow." Snoring and even bed-wetting may indicate the possible presence of sleep apnea. Childhood apnea is found more often in children who are overweight or who have enlarged tonsils and adenoids.

## Snoring

Spouses are often the ones who recognize their partners' sleep disorders, especially when loud snoring is involved. The noise can disrupt the sleep of anyone in earshot.

If you would like to quiet the noise of your snoring, try making a few simple changes in your lifestyle:

- Avoid alcohol after dinner.
- Don't take tranquilizers. (They relax the muscle

tone in your throat, lower your breathing, and increase your chances of apnea.)

∞ If you have a stuffy nose, take a decongestant. (Find one that does not list excitability or sleeplessness as a side effect, or try a nasal strip such as Breathe Right® to open your nasal passages. Other products, like Breathe Fit® and Breathe With Eez®, are reusable devices that fit inside your nose to widen airways.)

∞ Don't sleep on your back.

∞ Check out the possibility that obesity or large adenoids are contributing to the problem.

∞ Ask your doctor about somnaplasty, a thirty-minute outpatient procedure to open the breathing passage.

Remember that more than half of all heavy snorers have sleep apnea. If your snoring is a symptom of apnea, see the treatments in the sleep apnea section above.

## Restless Legs Syndrome

People who suffer from restless legs syndrome (RLS) might say, "My legs feel crawly" or "weird" or "jumpy." According to a report from Johns Hopkins Medical Center, these ill-defined sensations of deep-seated discomfort in the calves, or the jerky leg movements that occur when trying to fall asleep, occur in one out of seven people over fifty years of age. However, they have also been observed in children as young as four years old.

RLS occurs while awake, but it falls into the sleep-disorder category because it often prevents a person from falling asleep. It also interferes with the length of time RLS sufferers can sit still, thereby affecting their ability to travel comfortably, enjoy forms of entertainment that involve sitting for a period of time, and even attend business meetings. Its discomfort can last from ten minutes to several hours.

Theories vary on why RLS strikes, but it's comforting to note that it is not related to emotional or psychiatric disorders. RLS is a nerve disorder that some believe starts in childhood but doesn't cause symptoms until later in life, when circulation of blood in the legs becomes sluggish. It may result from low levels of dopamine, a chemical that helps transmit nerve impulses. Although restless legs may exist independently of other diseases, it occurs more often in pregnant women, older people, and those with such medical conditions as iron-deficiency anemia, rheumatoid arthritis, and diabetes. Dr. Samuel Dunkell, director of the Insomnia Medical Services in New York City, also notes that "there is a family incidence in 75 percent of the cases," suggesting that the majority of RLS cases are hereditary.[6]

To treat RLS, your physician may recommend Levodopa, a drug used for patients with Parkinson's disease that has also been used successfully for restless legs. Dopamine and natural vitamin E are also receiving praise for their effectiveness in treating RLS. Carbamazepine and Clonazepam, drugs usually reserved for seizure control, may also be prescribed, as might Lithium and antidepressants.

Below are several suggested remedies, some offered by professionals, others by RLS sufferers themselves:

- Move around frequently; stand up and stretch your legs.

- ❧ Try a leg massage to increase blood flow.

- ❧ Include a daily banana in your diet, along with six glasses of water each day.

- ❧ Avoid caffeine and eat less sugar.

- ❧ Ask your doctor about biofeedback. It helps eliminate the negative effects of stress by teaching a "relaxation response" during difficult times.

- ❧ Take antacid tablets.

- ❧ Take a warm bath before bed or use a heating pad on your legs. If heat doesn't help, try an ice pack.

- ❧ Sleep on a textured surface, like corduroy or wool; the fibers tend to soothe afflicted leg muscles.

Note that over-the-counter sleep medications seem to make restless legs syndrome worse.[7]

## Periodic Limb Movement

Periodic limb movement (PLM) is characterized by the involuntary jerking and/or twitching of legs (and sometimes arms) while sleeping. These jerks and twitches may last from a few minutes to several hours and are often strong enough to disrupt sleep many times a night. Fifty percent of sleepers affected by a mild form of this disorder are unaware they have it because they sleep through the episodes. Others, however, awaken continually and complain of nighttime insomnia and excessive drowsiness during the day. A person's spouse is often the key to recognizing the symptoms, as well as bed sheets that are in disarray by morning.

Most people with RLS experience some amount of periodic limb movements as well. However, those with periodic limb movements do not usually have restless legs syndrome.

While the causes of periodic limb movement remain a mystery, research has ruled out any association with seizures such as those caused by epilepsy. PLM may appear in conjunction with sleep apnea or nerve or muscle disorders. Certain medications (antidepressants, for example) might trigger it, as well as withdrawal from tranquilizers or sedatives. Poor circulation, kidney or liver disease, or anemia may also play a role, as can pregnancy or a back injury. It is found more often in women than men and becomes more common as people age.

Those who are awakened often by PLM can benefit from regular exercise, good nutrition, and behaviors that help improve sleep. If you take an antidepressant medication, you would probably benefit from changing to one that doesn't instigate leg movements. When required, physicians treat this disorder with Sinemet (a medication for sufferers of Parkinson's disease) or with vitamin and mineral supplements (especially vitamin E). They also recommend taking a warm bath before going to bed.

## Nocturnal Leg Cramps

Leg cramps differ from periodic leg movements in that they are not periodic, and the episodes usually last longer. Leg cramps wake up the sleeper with a painful contraction of the calf and foot muscles. They may be caused by a potassium, calcium, or magnesium deficiency, or by wearing shoes with high heels or little arch support. Many women experience them during pregnancy. Sciatic nerve problems can also cause them.

These cramps are usually relieved by a massage or by flexing your feet upward for several seconds or leaning forward against a wall while keeping your feet flat on the floor. If a deficiency is to blame, try taking a supplement to increase the mineral's level in your body. For an irritated sciatic nerve, you may need to use a prescribed inflammatory medication. Some people have found natural vitamin E to be particularly effective in easing leg cramps.

## Sleepwalking

The term *sleepwalking* covers a range of behaviors that take place in the night while a person is partly asleep and partly awake. The chemical "instruction" that usually keeps the body immobile while the brain sleeps doesn't "kick in," and the sleeper may wander around the house, eat, go outside, even drive. Contrary to the popular belief that sleepwalking is not dangerous, this practice *can* be life-threatening if the sleepwalker trips, falls down stairs, or drives a car without being fully awake and responsive. The person's eyes may be open, but he does not comprehend what he is seeing; his facial expression remains blank. It is not dangerous to awaken him, but he will probably be confused or disoriented if you do so.

The cause of sleepwalking in adults is usually linked to a high level of anxiety or some personality disturbance. No specific treatment is recommended for this disorder other than making sure the environment is safe by removing objects the sleeper might trip over. Those who are prone to sleepwalking should avoid alcohol and other central nervous system depressants. If necessary, a tranquilizer (like a benzodiazepine) may prove helpful.

## REM-Sleep Behavior Disorder

One night, Joanie woke to find her husband under their bed busily fussing with the box springs. Later, he told her he dreamed he was working on their car.

On another occasion, a patient in a sleep lab spent much of the night carefully tying invisible fishing flies, although his brain waves indicated he was sound asleep.

Both of these people exhibited mild forms of REM-sleep behavior disorder, which occurs mostly in middle-aged and older men. Such episodes happen during the dream phase of sleep when the body is mostly paralyzed. However, a sleeper with this disorder seems able to act out his dreams, often with violent behavior, such as kicking or punching. Though unconscious, he may prove dangerous to himself or another, responding to others as to an enemy. Once awakened, he will remember his dream, which is usually consistent with his actions while he was asleep.

If you or your spouse exhibits such behavior, contact your physician. Further occurrences can be suppressed when a drug treatment is instituted. (Clonazepam is one drug that is effective in treating this disorder.) In the meantime, make sure your bedroom is safety-proofed by removing lamps, tables, or anything else that might be used as a "weapon" by the sleeper.

## Tooth Grinding

My husband suffers from the grinding, gnashing, or clenching of teeth during sleep that characterizes *bruxism*. Fifteen percent of the population of the United States suffers from this malady, which usually occurs in the early-morning hours. It can be so forceful that it actually wears down the sleeper's teeth.

Bruxism may be caused by a malocclusion—the way a person's upper and lower jaws fit together—or psychological factors, such as suppressed tension, anger, or anxiety. Alcohol intake worsens the situation.

Treatment varies, depending on the specific situation. Wearing a plastic mouth guard, specially fitted by a dentist or orthodontist, is used if needed to protect the sleeper's teeth. Some individuals may need their bites readjusted, while others might benefit from psychotherapy to better manage stress and anger in their lives. Abstinence from alcohol is recommended for everyone who suffers from this affliction.

## Narcolepsy

Television sitcoms have found humor in a character's tendency to nod off at inappropriate times. However, such behavior may signify a genetic, neurological disorder called narcolepsy, which is characterized by irresistible sleepiness and uncontrollable urges to nap briefly throughout the day. Because of the way narcolepsy affects people's lives, it should be taken seriously and treated.

In addition to sleeping off and on during the day, narcoleptics have poor nighttime sleep patterns as well, falling almost directly into REM sleep instead of progressing through the NREM stages. Besides excessive daytime sleepiness and unpredictable naps (even while driving), a narcoleptic may exhibit *cataplexy*, in which intense emotions can weaken muscles so that the person may drop something or even fall down.

*Sleep paralysis* is another symptom of narcolepsy. This paralysis, which occurs either when falling asleep or waking up, is temporary but alarming. When this paralysis occurs, the sleeper feels unable to move. *Hypnogogic hallucinations* may also occur at sleep onset or awaking. These dreamlike experiences cause people to hear strange sounds or see imaginary figures in the room. *Automatic behavior* is also characteristic of narcolepsy. A person might act normally but not remember a certain period of time. This may be unnerving at best and dangerous at worst when it occurs, for example, while driving.

Heredity plays a role in narcolepsy, which usually begins when a person is quite young, but may not be noticeable for many years. It is relatively mild in the beginning; however, if it increases in severity without treatment, it may impair the person's ability to hold a job or maintain relationships.

The Multiple Sleep Latency Test (MSLT) is used to diagnose narcolepsy by measuring the amount of daytime sleepiness. The test is performed in a sleep lab, where the patient lies down in a darkened room and takes a series of naps at prescribed intervals. Polysomnography (EEG monitoring) measures the person's brain waves during sleep, as well as sleep-onset time. An early onset of the REM-sleep stage distinguishes narcolepsy from other sleep disorders.

Although there currently is no cure for narcolepsy, treatments are available to bring symptoms under control. Nondrug treatment involves a consistent bedtime and waking schedule, as well as short, scheduled naps to reduce the frequency of "sleep attacks."

Stimulants are often prescribed to keep patients alert, while antidepressants are used to suppress REM sleep, preventing cataplectic attacks. Ritalin, often prescribed for hyperactivity, is also used successfully with narcoleptics.

The American Narcolepsy Association and the Narcolepsy Network provide further information and can direct interested patients to a local support group.[8]

Before we leave this topic, remember that although the sleep disorders described in this chapter are the most prevalent nighttime maladies, they are only a small number of those that can affect a good night's sleep. If you believe you have a physical reason for your sleeplessness but the symptoms described above don't quite "fit," rest assured that a sleep specialist is usually able to diagnose sleep problems and treat them successfully. Don't hesitate to seek help.

# Chapter Six

# The Behavioral Connection

*Adjusting Your Lifestyle*

"Is there such a thing as a sleep makeover?" Jenny asked me as we had coffee. "I read about facial and hairstyle makeovers, but I know I'd feel like a new person if I could just get a real night's sleep!"

Well, there's good news, Jenny. We can often enhance our "sleepability" by a lifestyle "makeover"—making minor adjustments such as establishing a constant bedtime routine or cutting out that after-dinner cappuccino. Or we may need more significant modifications, like beginning a consistent exercise program or giving up cigarettes. Here are some practical suggestions of things that have worked for others. I hope they will help you too.

## Exercise

Americans have been called "couch potatoes," a term that reflects our sedentary lifestyles. Instead of engaging in vigorous activity, we sit in front of our television sets for hours. Add the presence of personal computers in our homes, and we've now become "mouse potatoes" as well. If this describes you, be encouraged that it's not too late to get moving. Besides relieving tension in our muscles and generally improving the well-being of body and mind, exercise is a crucial part of sleep fitness. If we insomniacs give our bodies a good workout during the day, we will be more relaxed and sleep-ready at night.

As you embark on an exercise program, keep in mind the following.

*Exercise vigorously.* Because aerobic exercise increases your metabolic and heart rates, leaving you feeling energized rather than sleepy, any strenuous workout should take place at least six hours before bedtime. Your body needs time to wind down before sleep will come.

*Start each workout with low intensity movements.* Gently stretch your muscles to warm them up and prevent injury. Cool down after each strenuous session with a sustained time of stretching to help you relax and prevent sore muscles. There are many helpful videos and books on the market to teach you safe and effective routines.

*Don't tire yourself out.* If you awake during the night, do not try to tire out your body by doing push-ups or the like. It won't work. Instead, do some gentle arm and leg stretches.

Note: Be sure to discuss any new exercise program with your physician before you begin.

## Relax

Relaxing is easier said than done, considering the stressful pace most of us keep these days. Yet there are many relaxation techniques so time-tested and varied that you can surely find one or two that will work for you.

*Breathe deeply and slowly.* When you concentrate on your breathing, your body responds in many positive ways. Deep breathing lessens fatigue, increases energy, relaxes tense muscles, and improves circulation.

To receive the full benefit of deep breathing, maintain good posture whether you are sitting, standing, or even lying down. Let your abdomen expand and contract as you inhale and exhale, and be sure to pause between breaths. Do this when you get up in the morning, again in the afternoon for renewed energy, then at night to alleviate the day's stress and prepare your body for sleep.

*Stretch those tense muscles.* Find a videocassette or take a class that demonstrates stretching techniques, specifically one designed for relaxation. A friend of mine, who began practicing yoga positions for greater flexibility, found that as an added benefit she felt more relaxed after these stretching exercises. You might also relax by taking an evening stroll to wind down after a busy day.

*Boost your sense of humor.* Laughter therapy is growing in popularity as people seek to approach life's challenges with lighthearted optimism. Their purpose is not to trivialize suffering but to help themselves and others through difficult situations by finding a humorous element. Some people notice that playing with children or a pet lifts their spirits. Others find humor by reading joke books, watching comedies, or spending more time with friends who have an upbeat disposition.

*Listen to music or other recordings to create a tranquil setting and block out distracting noises.* Select the forms of music you find most relaxing, or choose from recordings of gently falling rain, a mild breeze through the treetops, or neutral "white noise." Soothe your spirit by replacing the dissonant noises around you with musical or natural sounds. Some recordings are made specifically for sleep enhancement.

*Relax by listening to a book on audiocassette.* A friend of mine gets books-on-tape from the library. As she just listens, she finds herself able to rest her arms, shoulders, and even her eyes.

*Take a few "time-outs" throughout the day.* Carve out a minute or two every so often to look out the window, say a prayer, or even step outside for a breath of fresh air. Or try counting backwards from ten, pausing between each number to say, "Relax." When you reach number one, let all of your muscles grow heavy and loose. Remain that way for five minutes. Such brief activities will refresh you and help reduce stress in your mind and body.

Some people find help by turning to a chiropractor to help alleviate tension. "When people aren't managing their stress properly," says Stephen Dreier, D.C., "it often manifests itself as neck or back pain. They might sleep better from the relaxation response to an adjustment. We treat the whole person by teaching our patients relaxation techniques, behavior modification, posture, and how to handle changes in their environments."

## Take a Bath

We live in an age of efficiency, where we continually strive to make the best use of our time, money, and energy. Automatic washing machines long ago replaced labor-intensive wringer washers, which had already made hand-held washboards obsolete. Dishwashers have become a standard feature of the contemporary American home, and bathtubs often stand unused as we turn to the more expedient shower. Yet our modern conveniences have unwittingly "thrown out the baby with the bathwater." While eliminating the manual processes of cleaning our clothing, our dishes, and our bodies, their therapeutic effects have vanished as well.

The bath is returning to its place as an honored pre-bedtime ritual as people come to recognize its value as a sleep-inducer. Soaking in a tub full of warm water, unhurried, helps us unwind. Hydrotherapy— the therapeutic use of water—has come into its own as an important part of self-care.

More and more, bathrooms designed to welcome and envelop in comfort those who enter are show-cased in home-decorating magazines. You can create a peaceful atmosphere in your own bathroom by lighting one or more scented candles and playing soothing music as you enjoy a twenty- to thirty-minute soak in bath salts or oils. Search out the many bath products available today in department stores, pharmacies, and even shops exclusively devoted to "the bath." You might even want to build a collection by asking for these items as gifts for birthdays or other special occasions.

If this sounds too indulgent, too pricey, or too feminine, note that you needn't have the perfect color scheme, the thickest bath towels, or expensive bath salts to de-stress effectively. Simply dissolving a cup of Epsom or kitchen salt in a tub of comfortably hot water will provide the same benefits found in legendary mineral hot springs. As your muscles and joints relax, your mind will also. Because your body cools as it emerges from hot water, baths encourage our bodies to sink into sleep more easily.

Your skin dries out more quickly when you bathe regularly, so experts suggest you limit your long soaks to once a week. Even a hot shower can help your mind and body prepare for sleep. Follow up your bath by gently rubbing a moisturizer into your skin.

## Try a Massage

"We usually only touch ourselves when we hurt," Gayle Morrow, a certified massage therapist, maintains. "But touch is as essential as food and water. We need it at all ages, but the very young and the very old need it most, as well as those who are hurting." Morrow tells her clients to get in touch with their bodies, treat them carefully and gently, and they will learn what theirs needs most.

One of the best ways to release tension in your muscles is to get a professional therapeutic massage. In this treatment the therapist applies rhythmic kneading, smooth strokes, and concentrated pressure to calm the client's nerves, warm muscles, and release tension in the muscles. Other benefits usually include decreased soreness and fatigue, increased mobility, and increased circulation.

You may arrange for a licensed massage therapist to visit your home or go to his or her office for treatment. Professional therapists will ask you to complete a health questionnaire, customize treatment to your needs, and assure your privacy throughout the procedure, which can take from thirty to ninety minutes. Many therapists believe in the benefits of self-massage and can teach you effective techniques to use at home. You may find it enjoyable to take turns giving and receiving massages with a loved one.

If you prefer not to invest in a session with a personal therapist, here are a few techniques to try:

- ❧ Begin by getting comfortable, then gently rub wherever you hurt.

- ❧ Pinch carefully along the fleshy tops of your shoulders to relax the muscles.

- ❧ Sitting in a comfortable chair, cradle the back of your neck with your hands. Squeeze gently, slowly rolling your head in a circle. Release and repeat several times.

- ❧ Using your fingertips, press any areas in your neck, shoulders, head, hands, or feet that are sore or tense, moving in a circular, rhythmic motion.

- ❧ Ask your partner to press along the sides of your spine.

- ❧ Grasp a handful of hair, then gently pull it in a circular motion, moving the scalp below.

In addition to hands-on therapy, businesses today market a realm of devices designed to massage, heat, and vibrate aching muscles. Back and neck massagers, heat mittens, and magnetic insoles for your shoes are just a few of the products that exist to soothe what ails you.

## Watch Your Diet

Physician Diane Komp writes in her book *Breakfast for the Heart,* "There's a saying in German that stands in sharp contrast to modern eating habits: 'Eat the supper of a pauper, the midday meal of a burgher, and breakfast of a king.' This alimentary advice is a sensible path to a peaceful night's sleep."[1] The timing and types of food you eat before bedtime can help or hurt your ability to sleep well, so give careful thought to what you eat in the evening or in the middle of the night. Certain foods promote sleep; others do just the opposite.

A light snack prior to going to bed may help you relax, especially one heavy in carbohydrates such as bread, crackers, or a potato. Carbohydrates are processed quickly and help speed tryptophan, a sleep-inducing amino acid, to the brain. Such foods bring on sleep more quickly than those high in protein, which tend to increase alertness. Many people find that milk and other dairy products, rich in tryptophan, help them go to sleep faster. Warm milk is a traditional, time-tested favorite.

Avoid eating heavy or spicy foods just before bedtime. They create excess stomach acid, which may back up into the esophagus, causing indigestion and interfering with sleep. Also, stay away from foods that produce gas, such as beans and raw fruits and vegetables.

High-fat foods are harder to digest and sit heavier in your stomach than those with a lower fat content. Keep in mind that whatever you eat close to bedtime is more likely to be stored in your body as fat than food eaten earlier in the day.

Say yes to low-fat cereal, air-popped popcorn, bagels, English muffins, fig bars, graham crackers, fresh fruit, or frozen fruit or yogurt bars.

Say no to ice cream, cake, pizza, barbecue, nachos, beef, and full-fat cheeses.

Try to eat at night only when you are hungry, not because you are bored or worried. Overeating causes more problems than it solves. Drinking beverages before retiring causes some people to get up in the night to use the bathroom. If this describes you, try restricting your fluid intake before retiring.

## Cut Out Caffeine

Caffeine has become the drug of choice for a large number of people who would never consider taking an illegal drug. Yet caffeine is a powerful stimulant of the body's central nervous system, and if we drink coffee after dinner, it's no wonder we can't sleep.

Caffeine's stimulating effect reaches maximum concentration in the bloodstream about thirty minutes after it is ingested. Three hours later, it has only been half eliminated from our systems. Therefore experts suggest discontinuing caffeine at least four to six hours before bedtime. One man who suffered from back spasms at night due to arthritis in his spine found that caffeine triggered spasms as long as six hours later. Once he stopped consuming caffeine, his spasms disappeared.

Coffee is not the only source of caffeine in our diet. It is also present in chocolate, nonherbal teas (hot or iced), many soft drinks (particularly colas, but also some of the citrus-flavored, carbonated beverages), and even medications, especially allergy and cold remedies and some aspirin formulations. Read labels if you are caffeine-sensitive.

Each of us varies in our sensitivity to caffeine, and this seems to increase as we age. If you are a problem sleeper, it would be wise to substitute decaffeinated versions of your favorite beverages. Some people complain that even decaffeinated coffee keeps them awake, so you will have to discover what works best for you.

## Avoid Alcohol

Some people claim that a "nightcap" helps them relax and fall asleep, and this may be true. Alcohol—in contrast to caffeine—acts as a depressant in the central nervous system. However, while alcohol may induce sleep initially, its sedative effect wears off long before morning. In fact, as the body metabolizes alcohol, it releases a natural stimulant, which often leads to nighttime awakenings and lighter sleep. After awakening in the night, that person may have trouble getting back to sleep.

Chronic alcohol abuse causes more serious problems by creating abnormal sleep patterns. Alcohol-dependent individuals may have hundreds of awakenings each night and little deep sleep. Their sleep-wake rhythm is indistinct. They are excessively sleepy during the day, even when they spend a longer time in bed. In addition, alcohol triggers sleep apnea, up to five times more frequently than in people who do not consume alcohol.

When heavy drinkers stop drinking, their insomnia may increase at first, but their sleep will usually begin to improve in about two weeks. However, in some cases it may take years to return to normal.

Never mix alcohol and sleeping pills. Combining them can lead to serious side effects and may even prove fatal.

## Stop Smoking

Added to the other health risks of smoking, nicotine stimulates the central nervous system and thus interferes with sleep. In spite of the sense of relaxation some experience, as the amount of nicotine entering the body increases, so do its detrimental side effects: increased heart rate, blood pressure, and brain-wave activity.

Laboratory studies have traced the association of sleep difficulties with ingested nicotine. Smokers usually take longer to fall asleep, and they wake up more frequently than nonsmokers. Smoking before bedtime also contributes to frequent nighttime awakenings.

Clearly, quitting smoking improves sleep quality even as it reduces the risk of lung cancer and other diseases. If you have tried to quit but cannot, try to decrease the amount of nicotine you put into your system prior to bedtime.

## Bring Order to Your Day

Days filled with chaos, crises, and confusion give rise to turbulent nights. Despite the fact that occasionally situations arise that are beyond our control, we can generally bring some regularity to our daily activities. Our bodies function best within some sort of routine, even if we can't always maintain it perfectly.

Jerry found this out the hard way. Two years ago his life seemed to be always teetering on the edge of catastrophe. He felt pulled in different directions by the needs of his family, his real estate clients, his church, and the various associations and community groups to which he belonged. Rarely did he enjoy a meal without being interrupted by his ever-present cellular phone. At work he found himself preoccupied by concerns at home, and vice versa. His mind never stopped working, and this affected his sleep as well as the relationships in his life.

Unfortunately for Jerry, it took a heart attack at age forty-three to make him sit back and review his life.

As he recovered from bypass surgery, he thought about who and what were most important to him, then outlined a reasonable schedule to reflect his newly recognized priorities. He began slowly to give greater consideration to time management. Jerry was pleased to discover that becoming more proactive about his use of time during the day led to his sleeping better at night.

If your days seem out of control, pushed and shoved by others' demands and an overcommitted schedule, take a break and reevaluate how well you manage your time. You probably can't change everything at once, but at least make a start. If possible, begin getting up and going to bed at the same times each day. Establish some regular times with your family to sit down and enjoy meals and conversation together. Get regular exercise and take some time to relax each day. Your body will appreciate it and reward you with better sleep.

## Do Something for Someone Else

For those with chronic problems such as pain or insomnia, it is easy to become self-focused and exhausted with the effort of coping. Ironically, when we turn our attention and energy outward and begin to practice acts of kindness toward other people, our own difficulties seem less overwhelming.

The Bible gives us some help here: "Let us not become weary in doing good, for at the proper time we will reap a harvest if we do not give up. Therefore, as we have opportunity, let us do good to all people" (Galatians 6:9-10). And another verse encourages us to "see how inventive we can be in encouraging love and helping out" (Hebrews 10:24, *The Message*).

If you find yourself sighing with fatigue instead of inspiration, you are not alone. However, I believe that God calls us to do only what he will empower us to do. A verse I try to remember each day reads: "I can do everything through him who gives me strength" (Philippians 4:13). No matter how tired we are, we always feel better after we have done something for someone who needed our help or offered a word of encouragement or a listening ear.

The self-help techniques discussed above are most effective after a treatable physical condition has been ruled out. If these behavior modification methods don't help you get to sleep faster or stay asleep longer, seek a professional diagnosis of your sleeplessness.

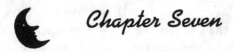

*Chapter Seven*

# The Day-Night Connection

*Resetting Your Internal Clock*

"God separated the light from the darkness. . . . And there was evening, and there was morning—the first day" (Genesis 1:4-5). Since the beginning, our planet has operated in cycles of light and darkness. We measure these cycles of time with a twenty-four-hour clock. But what happens when our internal "body clocks" have gotten out of sync with our world? What do we do when insomnia has upset our normal sleep-wake rhythm? When our jobs require a different pattern of getting up and going to bed than when the sun rises and sets? When jet lag throws off our schedule, and we just can't seem to get back on track?

## Circadian Rhythms

Our body clock controls when we are ready to sleep and when we're ready to wake up. The schedule on which our bodies operate—our circadian rhythm—reflects nature's timetable. Yet our individual, internal timing mechanisms often operate on a sleep-wake cycle that varies somewhat from a perfect twenty-four-hour day. In fact, the word *circadian* refers to any cycle that recurs approximately every twenty-four hours. Most people's body rhythms extend somewhat beyond that, some by more than sixty minutes. These cycles tend to be longer when we are young, decreasing as we age. Without the restrictions placed on us by our culture, clocks, and commitments, many of us would probably go to bed later and later each successive night and get up later and later each morning.

Scientists believe that an individual's circadian system is largely determined by genetics and our body's aging process.[1] The circadian rhythms of body temperature, hormonal changes, and sleep-wake schedules are coordinated at the base of our brains. A pathway runs from this part of the brain to our eyes, which explains why light seems to have such a significant effect on when we become alert or drowsy. Our body temperatures rise in our final hours of sleep, helping us to wake up more alert. They drop in the afternoon, accounting for early-afternoon sleepiness.

Our body's unique ability to respond to nature's time cues and society's demands often leads to internal conflict and disturbed sleep cycles. For example, when we are exposed to indoor lighting after sunset, our internal clocks are reset so that our peak demand for sleep occurs at about 4:00 A.M. instead of closer to midnight, as would occur without exposure to artificial light.

To maintain a regular schedule, our bodies need consistent information about light and darkness. Light-therapy treatments, which regulate our sleep-wake timetable, include the following:

- ❧ Dim the lights in the evening.
- ❧ Go to bed and get up at the same time every day of the week.

❧ Avoid artificial light after your regular bedtime hour.

❧ Sleep in a dark room.

❧ Wake up to bright light in the morning.

## The Nap Controversy

Should we or shouldn't we take time out for a snooze in the middle of the day? If so, when and for how long? If not, why not? Let's look at these questions as they affect both a regular nap and an occasional nap.

People who live in cultures that schedule post-lunchtime "siestas" take naps on a regular basis. If your schedule permits a daily nap, go ahead and allow yourself a short snooze in the early afternoon *as long as it doesn't interfere with your night's rest.* Insomniacs must be especially cautious not to abuse daytime dozing.

Naps can recharge your brain during its midday "circadian trough," the sleepy state that hits between noon and 4:00 P.M. each day. Nap researcher David Dinges, chief of sleep and chronobiology in the psychiatry department of the University of Pennsylvania, says that even brief periods of daytime sleep can increase people's alertness and performance levels, as well as make them feel more refreshed. Twenty-minute periods of sleep are usually adequate, Dinges says.[2]

Psychologist Timothy Roehrs disagrees with the benefits of short naps; he advocates napping at least half an hour. Having studied the association between nap length and alertness at the Henry Ford Hospital's Sleep Disorders Research Center in Detroit, Roehrs says that people need at least thirty minutes to significantly raise their mental sharpness. In fact, an hour would more closely mirror the pattern of a good night's sleep, he says, when the sleeper has time to cycle through all the sleep stages.[3]

The timing of your nap is also an important consideration. Roehrs says most people can drop off more quickly and sleep more deeply between noon and 2:00 P.M. He advises people to use that time to catch up after a sleepless night.

Most sleep specialists agree that nappers should never sleep more than two hours in the daytime. Long naps have a negative impact on natural sleep-wake rhythms, and post-nap grogginess affects the rest of the day.

## Mood Swings

"Some hours of the day, we're happier than others, and it's occurring inside of us, not just in reaction to the world around us," declares David Dinges. According to two recent studies done in Boston and Manchester, England, we can significantly influence our moods by changing the times when we wake and when we sleep.

Even if we have gotten enough sleep, we might be irritable or sad if our waking hours coincide with a time when our biological clock tells us we "should" be asleep. We could be extremely sleep-deprived, yet feel great during a time when our bodies say it's time to be awake.

Most of us do not usually control when we sleep and when we wake. Any number of circumstances may cause our body rhythms to malfunction, producing circadian-rhythm disorders. While we can regulate some of these, we must learn how to adapt to others.

## Sunday-Night Insomnia

Ken experienced what is commonly known as "Sunday-night insomnia." His weekend pattern was to stay up later than usual on Friday night, then sleep in on Saturday morning. He usually stayed up late again on Saturday night, then slept longer on Sunday morning. If he got up to go to church instead of sleeping in, he would take a long afternoon nap to make up for the sleep he had lost the night before. By Sunday night he couldn't get to sleep at the normal time.

If you regularly have difficulty falling asleep on Sunday nights and your weekend schedule is similar to Ken's, try to maintain a more regular schedule throughout the entire week. Go to bed at the same time every night, weekend or not. Forego a Sunday afternoon nap, and see if it helps. Sunday night insomnia is often corrected easily because it is due simply to a temporary shift in your sleep-wake rhythm.

## Jet Lag

Diana and Gary were excited about their first trip to Europe. They obtained passports, made reservations, changed their currency, and packed with anticipation. Their flight went well, and upon landing they set off to explore all the places they had looked forward to seeing in their two-week stay. However, even before the end of the first day, they found their energy diminishing. Both had trouble sleeping the first several nights, and they both felt irritable during the days. "Our friends love their trips here." Diana shook her head. "What's our problem?"

Traveling across time zones disrupts the body's biological rhythms and causes a condition known as "jet lag." This widely experienced circadian problem is characterized by various physiological and psychological effects—sleeplessness at night, daytime sluggishness, indigestion, irritability, and poor concentration. These effects can last for more than a week, until the traveler adjusts to the time cues of the new environment. (Even if we don't travel, many of us experience a mild sense of jet lag twice a year when we switch to and from daylight-saving time.)

Experts suggest the following tips for coping with jet lag.

1. Select a flight that arrives in the early evening, then stay up until 10:00 P.M. local time.

2. Discover the use of bright light to reset your biological clock. For example, when you fly westward, expose yourself to bright light in the late afternoon. This will enable you to stay up later at your destination. When you fly eastward, get plenty of bright morning light to advance your body's rhythms.

3. When you pack, think about your sleep needs. Include earplugs, eye shades, and anything else you think could help minimize the distractions of an unfamiliar place.

4. Drink water or juices en route to your destination, because dehydration inhibits your body's ability to adjust its rhythms. Avoid alcohol and overeating, and try to get some light exercise as you travel.

5. Allow yourself extra time to adjust to the new schedule. When you fly westward, start getting up and going to bed later several days before your flight. When going east, begin getting up and going to bed earlier. Once you arrive, plan for extra rest, perhaps taking a short nap each day until you adapt to the new time zone.

6. If all else fails, try a short-acting sleeping pill

prescribed by your physician to use for no more than three to four weeks, because it will lose its effectiveness after that time.

7. Ask your doctor about melatonin, a substance that occurs naturally in the body and increases in the bloodstream at night. Some studies suggest that taking melatonin at prescribed times helps promote sleep onset. Many scientists urge caution about the use of melatonin because the studies done thus far have produced contradictory results; some are concerned about possible adverse effects not yet observed; and, because melatonin is not regulated like drugs, product purity is not assured.[4]

## Shift Work

About one-fifth of the employees in the United States work nontraditional hours, such as nights or rotating shifts. Police officers, factory workers, air-traffic controllers, hospital personnel, truck drivers, and others find that sleep is challenging, even elusive.

Tom took a new job that requires him to work nights and is having trouble adjusting. Working at night requires that he try to sleep while his family and others around him are awake, then trying to work while they sleep. His sleep is often disrupted by sunlight, noise, and the warmer daytime temperatures.

When Cherie first started working as a nurse, she found it easy to accommodate her shifts in schedule as they occurred. However, after she got married and started a family, continuously adjusting her schedule to meet her family's needs became more and more difficult.

Like others who work rotating shifts, Cherie had to adjust to a new work schedule every few days. Her constantly changing sleep schedule forced her to sleep when activities around her—not to mention her own biological rhythms—told her she should be awake. A recent study shows that shift workers are two to five times more likely to fall asleep on the job than employees with regular, daytime hours. On average, shift workers get five to seven hours less sleep than they need during their work week. In addition, they often try to maintain a "normal" weekend schedule for their family's benefit.

Shift workers report greater fatigue and higher stress levels than "regular" workers. They are at greater risk for certain health problems, such as heart disease, gastrointestinal disorders, and menstrual dysfunction, and are more prone to on-the-job accidents. Research shows that truck drivers have more accidents during their biological clocks' "sleeping time," and sleep deprived doctors make mistakes more often than well-rested physicians.[5]

How do people like Tom and Cherie reconcile their sleep/work schedules with their environments, their families, and even their own bodies? The American Sleep Disorders Association advises:

- On the last few days of your evening shift, delay your bedtime and the time you get up by one to two hours. As the night shift begins, you will already be adapting to your new schedule.

- Allow for times of extra rest during your shift change, to help your body ease into your new schedule. Some companies allow their employees a week off between shift changes so their bodies can make the adjustment.

- Ask your doctor about the occasional use of a

short-acting sleeping pill to reduce the problems associated with changing sleep-wake rhythms.

It might also be helpful to drink caffeine only at the *beginning* of your shift, so you will be able to sleep when your shift ends. Then make sure you have a comfortable bed, room-darkening window-coverings, earplugs or a white-noise machine to block outside noise, if necessary. If you still have difficulty sleeping according to your unique schedule, ask your doctor for other steps you might take.

## Delayed Sleep Phase Syndrome

"I'm afraid I'm going to lose my job!" Trisha, age twenty-three, blurted out. "I try to go to bed around 10:30, but I'm a night owl by nature. I never can get to sleep until two or three in the morning. Then I sleep through my alarm and am late to work. What's going on? Why can't I get to sleep?"

Trisha could be experiencing the disorder known as delayed sleep phase syndrome (DSPS). It is more common in young adults, but even older people often struggle with its trauma. When it interferes with day-time responsibilities and relationships, it may indeed lead to loss of employment, poor grades, or high levels of stress.

Chronotherapy and light therapy are often helpful in treating this condition. (See next page.)

## Advanced Sleep Phase Syndrome

Advanced sleep phase syndrome, as distinct from delayed sleep phase syndrome, is more common among older adults, whose sleepiness begins in the early afternoon. When people's body clocks run faster than the twenty-four-hour day, they get sleepy as early as afternoon, fall asleep early in the evening, and awaken too early, unable to get back to sleep. Like those with delayed phase problems, a lack of sleep has little effect on the problem. No matter how late they remain awake in the evening, they continue to awaken very early the next morning.

## Treating Circadian Phase Disorders

Sometimes an abnormal sleep cycle is a symptom of depression or poor sleep habits. A professional evaluation usually leads to proper treatment.

*Light therapy* and *chronotherapy* are both effective in resetting body clocks. In light therapy, a person is exposed to bright light at certain times of the day to move the sleep cycle forward or back to achieve the desired effect. Chronotherapy moves a person's bedtime later and later until it has rotated to the desired bedtime and rescheduled the rhythms.

Melatonin, as mentioned above, has been called the "all-natural nightcap." A hormone secreted by the pineal gland during the night, it appears to regulate our sleep-wake cycles. Studies suggest that low doses of melatonin can hasten sleep without the side effects of sleeping pills. So far its most successful use has been to treat travelers with jet lag, as well as those suffering from mild sleep disorders. Unfortunately, it usually produces only a light sleep and so does not supply the benefits available to those who sleep deeply.

Although melatonin is generally considered safe, the recommended dose varies from individual to individual. Therefore I suggest using it only under a doctor's care. And because melatonin as a supplement is still in the experimental stage, women who are pregnant or nursing are advised to refrain from taking it, because of its unknown effect on babies.

Thomas Edison couldn't have foreseen the consequences his electric lightbulb would have on the sleeping habits of a nation. We have paid dearly for the privilege of electric light, sacrificing much-needed hours of sleep. The same technology that allows us to work and play long after sunset also disrupts many people's internal body clocks. Let's look at some additional preparations for sleeping that will help us adjust.

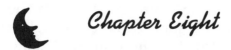 

# Chapter Eight

# The Environmental Connection

*Setting the Stage for Sleep*

To achieve the best sleep possible, we do well to create a quiet resting place, a haven where we can return regularly to be refreshed. When the goal is to set the stage for sleep, we need to check our environment for any potential trouble spots.

According to a recent survey of 1,000 adults, 26 percent reported that their sleep is frequently sabotaged by environmental factors.[1] Often the key to how well we sleep on a given night depends on our physical comfort level. The suitability and comfort of our bed, the room temperature, lighting, noise level, and even our bedroom's decor, along with how safe we feel all play important roles in our ability to fall asleep and stay asleep.

## Guard Your Bedroom

Let's take a tour of the room where you sleep. Seeing your familiar setting from a fresh perspective will give you greater creativity in solving your sleep problems.

Is that a desk in the corner covered with lots of papers—bills to write, correspondence to catch up on? I'm sure that's restful to see every night as you climb into bed. How's your mattress holding out? Lasted fifteen years, you say? Nice big TV there, too. And I see a bright red alarm clock next to your bed. Great for watching the minutes tick by as you lie awake at night.

Sleep experts say your bedroom should be reserved for only two things: sleep and sex. When you allow yourself to watch television, eat, work, or read in your bedroom, you tend to lose focus of the room's main purpose. Stimuli-sensitive individuals, in particular, need to guard it as a place dedicated to sleep.

Do whatever you can to create an inviting and sleep-friendly environment. Decorate with the colors you find most soothing—for example, a neutral beige, a dusty blue, or a cool green. Keep in mind that cooler colors and darker furnishings absorb light better than bright ones. This is especially important for those who need total darkness to fall asleep. It also helps to keep your room neat and clean to give yourself a sense of order and serenity.

## The Bed Factor

Probably the single most important factor in getting a really good night's sleep is the bed you sleep in. Osteopath Michael Van Straten observes:

> I am constantly amazed by how many people buy a bed when they get married and are still sleeping in the same one twenty years later. In that period the average family has changed its car seven times, the television three times, the refrigerator twice, the washing machine twice, the living-

room furniture at least once, the lawn mower often, and yet they stick to the same sagging, lumpy bed. . . . If you can't afford to change your bed, then at least put a sheet of plywood under the mattress.[2]

If you are uncomfortable on your current bed, check the condition of your mattress. Is it old and worn? A sleep set that is used frequently will wear out more quickly than one set aside for occasional guests, as will one that is used by a heavy individual or more than one person. As your body or lifestyle changes, the same kind of mattress you once found comfortable may no longer provide you with the rest you need. Also, according to the Better Sleep Council, technological advances and medical developments have improved the engineering of mattress and foundation construction, so that a mattress set you purchase today will be different than one you bought just ten years ago.[3]

Make sure your bed is large enough for comfort and that you have adequate room to move around, especially if you share a bed. Depending on how active a sleeper you or your spouse is, you may need to invest in a king-size bed or even use separate beds for sleeping.

Over the centuries people have slept successfully on all kinds of surfaces—hard and soft, horizontal and inclined. Experiment to see what works best for you. Does sleep come easier on a foam or innerspring mattress? You may find a waterbed most comfortable or that a bed board under your mattress gives needed back support.

If you choose an innerspring mattress, be sure to turn and rotate it regularly so it will wear evenly.

Rotate your foundation (e.g., box springs) as well. Some swear by a sheep's wool mattress pad, others by an egg-crate-like foam pad to cushion pressure points and reduce pain. Hospitals often use these to prevent pressure sores.

The number of sleeping pillows you use and their level of firmness make a difference as well. This is an individual preference. A friend of mine in college used no pillow, convinced that this gave her better posture and did not interfere with her sleeping comfort. I, on the other hand, faithfully tote my own pillow wherever I go, if I hope to get any sleep at all. My husband uses a contoured pillow to avoid neck pain. Pregnant women often use full-length "body pillows" to help cushion their changing body shapes. People with sinus or respiratory problems often find that using additional pillows or an elevated mattress helps them breathe more easily.

Choosing a pillow's content (down or polyester fiberfill) will depend on which you find most comfortable and whether you have allergies. The Hong Kong Hotel currently offers ten different specialty pillows to its guests, each type of pillow with a specific purpose, ranging from reducing snoring to supporting neck-curve variations to allowing air circulation for easier breathing and sleeping.

Your bed linens and nightwear should be fresh and not scratchy. Make sure that whatever you wear to bed fits loosely, allowing free movement to turn over and stretch your legs.

## Steady Room Temperature

Whether you keep your bedroom hot or cold, dry or humid, also depends on individual taste. Some people enjoy open windows and fresh air, while others prefer a more closed environment, especially if they are sensitive to noise or allergens. In any case, it's best to avoid extremes and keep your room well ventilated.

Remember that cooler temperatures are more conducive to sleep than warmer ones. Experts say that temperatures above 70 degrees Fahrenheit adversely affect sleep quality, while temperatures between 64 and 68 degrees seem to cause the least amount of sleep disruption.

## Dim the Lights

Scientists have discovered that 80 percent of a person's incoming sensory information is delivered visually by light and that our day-night rhythms are dramatically affected by cycles of light and darkness. Those cycles determine when we are most active and when we are most inclined to rest.

Children often find night-lights reassuring in the dark, but some adults (myself included) find that even a small amount of light keeps them awake. If you are especially sensitive to light, you may want to wear a sleep mask or install dark curtains or blinds over the windows to keep out stray rays or even a diffused brightness.

If you choose to leave your bed when you awaken in the night, avoid turning on a bright light. Intense light stimulates your brain and thereby disturbs your body's rhythm of light and darkness, which may lead to continued wakefulness.

## Drown Out Noise

Sensitivity to noise is a common problem for non-sleepers. While a continuous sound, such as the hum of an air conditioner, may not prove disruptive, sudden loud noises arouse even sound sleepers. The neighbor's barking dog, your snoring spouse, a loud crash of thunder—these noises can disrupt an otherwise good night's sleep. So what can you do?

First, insulate the room you sleep in with carpet, wallpaper, and draperies that will absorb, or at least muffle, sound. Keep your windows closed at night to make your room more soundproof. Try wearing earplugs. Screen out noise with the steady, low-level sound of white noise (experts have designed machines specifically for this purpose), or mask outside sounds by playing your radio at low volume. My younger daughter runs a fan all night during the summer to cover sporadic noises that are more audible when she leaves windows and doors open for better air movement.

## The Clock

In this age of digital timekeepers, a clock's annoying ticking rarely presents the problem it did in the past. However, for those who keep one eye on the clock at night, watching each illuminated minute dissolve into the next, anxiety increases when sleep doesn't come. If you are one of these people, experts advise you to hide your clock. Dr. Peter Hauri says that a bedroom should be "a time-free environment."

For a few of us, however, not being able to see the clock can produce even greater anxiety. If we awaken, say, to go to the bathroom, we may wonder if there is enough time to make it worth trying to go back to sleep. Rather than continually estimating what time it is, it's better to have a clock in view—if we promise ourselves not to look too often!

## Safe and Secure

To sleep soundly, make your bedroom a safe haven from the outside world. If you feel threatened when you go to bed, consider investing in more secure door locks and/or alarm systems to wake you in case of fire, an intruder, or whatever causes you anxiety. When I was single and living alone, a bedside telephone calmed my fears because I knew it was close by in case of an emergency.

Ultimately, however, our best and truest security comes from God, as King David learned when he faced nights surrounded by enemies eager to kill him. On one occasion he prayed these words: "I lie down and sleep; I wake again, because the LORD sustains me. I will not fear the tens of thousands drawn up against me on every side" (Psalm 3:5-6). His confidence lay in God's power to protect him. Some people keep a Bible at their bedside to remind them of their true source of security.

## When You're Away From Home

There come times in our lives when we are required to sleep in settings beyond our control. For example, when traveling on vacation or for business we may need to sleep in a motel, in someone else's home, or even in a tent. If you—like many sleep strugglers—find sleeping away from home difficult, do whatever you can, however small, to create an atmosphere that will attract sleep.

Recently, some motels have responded to travelers' need for a good night's sleep. For example, in cooperation with the National Sleep Foundation, Hilton Hotels surveyed their clientele to discover what they felt was needed for a restful night. Most people asked for quieter rooms, followed by better beds. Hilton Hotels responded by making "Sleep-Tight Rooms" available on request at five locations participating in the pilot project. These rooms are soundproofed and fitted with firm mattresses, heavy drapes, and minibars that serve decaffeinated beverages and no high-energy foods. They include miscellaneous gadgets such as face masks, earplugs, clock-lamps that increase a soft glow of light to wake guests thirty minutes before their designated wake-up time, and compact disc players that mimic noises of everything from a seashore to white noise.

Perhaps your current environment isn't designed to increase your "sleepability." Maybe you are reading this book in a hospital room, one of the most difficult places to get a good night's sleep. While most patients need a restful setting, they are awakened often by the taking of vital signs and by lights, bells, and voices. Long-term patients in particular need to somehow squeeze in necessary sleep-time to heal.

Or you may be awake and alone in a cheerless prison cell. Take your cue from two people in the Bible who created ways to make their environments more comfortable. For example, the apostle Paul wrote to his friend Timothy from prison, and asked him to bring his cloak and some reading material—small comforts for his cold, damp cell. In the Old Testament, when Joseph found himself in prison, he developed relationships with his guard and his fellow prisoners, making his surroundings more bearable.

Maybe your limited financial resources prevent you from carrying out some of the suggestions discussed above. Wherever you are, look for creative, even small ways to comfort both your body and mind. You'll sleep better for it.

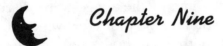 *Chapter Nine*

# The Psychological Connection

*Insomnia's Emotional Causes*

"I wouldn't lose sleep over it," the doctor told me after looking at my test results. "It doesn't look serious. We'll check it again in six months."

Easy for him to say. Unfortunately, just hearing those words made me anxious. And I know I'm not alone. Despite others' good intentions, we often lose precious hours of rest to the greedy monster of worry; a monster we can do without, especially if we already are prone to sleeplessness.

Other emotional monsters—fear, grief, depression, and anger—lurk in the shadows as well. Add to these the fast pace of our modern lifestyles, and the pressure skyrockets. This sets the scene for insomnia's arrival. In fact, many physicians say insomnia is the second most common complaint among their patients, after headaches.

"We live in a crazy world in which fear and insecurity are virtually universal experiences," says author Keith Miller. "The stress of our overcommitted lives often overflows into the nights and hinders our sleep." This stress, according to Miller, is "a silent but debilitating bedfellow."

What can we do to overcome the emotional toll that stress takes on our lives? We have looked at changing our attitudes toward insomnia and explored some physical aspects of the problem. We have considered ways to make our lifestyles and environments more conducive to sleep. Now it is time to examine the emotional baggage we bring with us to bed at night—and how we might set it aside so we can get our needed rest.

## Worry and Anxiety

"Sleep . . . knits up the ravelled sleeve of care." These words of William Shakespeare touch the hearts of those whose sleep is often buffeted by worry. "Sleep on it," he is saying, "and things will look better in the morning." If only we *could* sleep on it! There are two major types of worrying that keep a lot of us awake: anxiety and fear.

Anxiety is one of sleep's foremost foes. Seventy-four percent of one group of poor sleepers reported that they first encountered insomnia during a time of considerable stress.[1]

Countless numbers of us are anxious over how our needs will be met today, next year, or ten years down the road. The direction our concerns take usually depends on our life situation. People who struggle to find food, shelter, and clothing for each day worry over securing life's basic necessities. Those who live in comfortable homes with plenty of food and large wardrobes might worry about stock portfolios, corporate takeovers, and paying for their children's education.

In addition, our emotional world naturally turns upside-down when we lose a loved one, discover we have an inoperable illness, or suddenly find ourselves unemployed.

Simply responding to the pressures of everyday life is enough to overwhelm us with anxiety. And yet, we do not have to move through life feeling defeated or under attack. When we find ourselves burdened by cares and wide awake, we need to find ways to lift the load so sleep can squeeze its way in.

One way to banish anxiety is to just say no to your worries. Refuse to let them defeat you by setting them aside until you are better able to cope with them. Of course, I realize this is easier said than done. I've learned that by experience. For me, the most effective way to say no to worries is to pray, giving my concerns over to God, who is best able to do something about them. In doing so, I find relief, and I believe you can too. Jesus promised to help us do this: "Come to me, all you who are weary and burdened, and I will give you rest" (Matthew 11:28).

Sometimes I get up and write about whatever is bothering me. When I see my concerns on paper, it allows me to let them go until tomorrow.

For unfounded, excessive worry that lasts six months or more, fretful insomniacs would do well to talk things over with a trained counselor or physician. By visiting her doctor, Susan learned that her anxiety resulted from a chemical reaction in her brain. Since she began taking prescribed antianxiety medication, her ability to cope has improved considerably.

## Fear

Fear, an emotion so closely linked to anxiety that it's

difficult to discern the difference, is that knot-in-your-stomach feeling of apprehension you often take to bed with you. Burdensome by day, it feels even heavier at night, bearing down when you are most vulnerable. Whether fear is a vague foreboding or an awareness of a specific danger, your weary soul slumps under its weight.

Fear activates your fight-or-flight response to danger, real or imagined, and speeds adrenaline through your body, enabling you to confront or escape your enemy. Sleep retreats in deference to this stronger, more immediate force charging into the dark arena where you lie.

We fight many fears—fears of failure, of pain and suffering, of the future, of death, of losing jobs, relationships, loved ones, or financial security. Fear prevents us from trying new things, from developing new relationships.

The Bible encourages us to look to God to find freedom from fear. The psalmist David faced numerous threats to his safety, and many of his psalms reflect his fears under frightful circumstances. We see his faith triumph in verses such as Psalm 4:8: "I will lie down and sleep in peace, for you alone, O LORD, make me dwell in safety." Years later, the Old Testament prophet Zephaniah wrote this "lullaby":

> The LORD your God is with you,
>    he is mighty to save.
> He will take great delight in you,
>    he will quiet you with his love,
>    he will rejoice over you with singing.

The Bible speaks to our fears and anxieties with words of hope, wisdom, reassurance, and instruction. God promises to give us his power, through Christ, to defeat our foes, whether external or of our own making. So when the world and its worries turn up the heat in your life and keep you awake, I encourage you to drink deeply from God's waters of refreshment and find healing.

# Grief

My mother-in-law's doctor prescribed a short-term dose of sleeping pills to help her through the first few weeks following my father-in-law's sudden death. When someone we love dies, sleep often becomes the next fatality. We must not hesitate to seek medical intervention to help us get the physical rest we need to make it through those early days of fresh grief.

But after those days pass, how do we find rest?

The pain of loss visits us most vividly in the quiet darkness of night. Undistracted by the demands of the day, our minds can fill with memories and intensify our anguish. C. S. Lewis spoke from such an experience in his book *A Grief Observed,* after the death of his wife: "Her absence is like the sky, spread over everything." As we grieve, our bodies often leave us sleepless.

In the dark night of loneliness we turn inward, and some of us isolate ourselves. However, healing often comes through community, as others walk with us through our pain. It's not always easy, but we should allow those who offer comfort and practical care to minister to us. They can help keep us from despair.

Then, as soon as we can muster some bit of energy, we do well to reach out to others who are hurting, too. When we extend ourselves on behalf of others who suffer, we benefit as well. The prophet Isaiah wrote that when we share our food with the hungry, give shelter to the homeless, and clothe the naked, our "light will break forth like the dawn, and [our] healing will quickly appear" (Isaiah 58:8).

We can use our wakeful hours to pray. When we can't find the words, we can read some of the prayers in the book of Psalms. The psalmists expressed so well the sorrow in their lives, and they turned it toward God. We can make their words our own as we look to God for comfort and direction.

An understanding counselor, pastor, or priest is a valuable resource in times of great need. Make an appointment with one if your load becomes too heavy to bear alone.

## Depression

If you consistently wake up several hours earlier than you want to, it is often a sign of depression. Check the list on pages 32–33 to see if you have any other symptoms of depression—lost appetite, feelings of inadequacy, dark thoughts. Five or more affirmative answers suggests a strong probability of insomnia. Once you conquer your depression, your insomnia may disappear as well.

Since depression feeds on a vague sense of unease, many sufferers find that journaling allows them to investigate and articulate what they are feeling. Try it for yourself: Write out your emotions, filling three pages without worrying about how you express your thoughts in words. It's not for publication; it's therapy! This helps you explore your deepest emotions and often begin to see them in a different light. It's an act that releases tension.

Laughter, along with a positive attitude, can heal as well. Several recent studies have determined that, together, these can lead people to take better care of themselves and thus feel better. Whereas negative emotional states contract blood vessels and promote heart disease, laughter pumps the heart, exercises muscles, stimulates the brain, ventilates lungs, and raises the heart rate. People who make laughter part of their lives are better able to keep their perspective and restrain the negative emotions that contribute to bad habits. According to a study at Duke University, men and women who experienced depression, despair, and low self-esteem had a 70 percent greater risk of having a heart attack than those with a more positive perspective.

You may have to pretend good humor for a time. There is nothing wrong with that. Your body can't tell the difference between the physical reaction of a real or forced laugh and you will benefit just the same. In fact, you might be surprised at how soon you will find yourself in genuinely better spirits, just by "practicing."

Like persistent anxiety, severe depression is best treated by professionals. Don't hesitate to talk to your doctor or see a counselor for help in conquering this debilitating illness.

## Anger

"I'm sorry!" my daughter shouted after I told her to apologize to her sister.

"I forgive you," her sister replied in a syrupy, sing-song voice.

Despite their obvious insincerity, the girls soon ended their spat. Children forgive and forget far more quickly than we grown-ups do. Adults' superficial apologies and empty assurances of forgiveness are often harder to discern and leave disturbing matters unresolved.

The pressures of daily life often multiply until, at the end of the day when we are least able to cope, emotional molehills grow into overwhelming mountains. Petty grievances escalate. An ill-considered word can leave us fuming and isolated. If we are unsettled and tense at night because we are angry with someone—whether spouse, friend, or co-worker—we are probably damaging our own peace of mind far more than we are hurting the other person. Even if our anger is warranted, it can consume us.

Until we forgive, our anger allows us no rest. Until there is true forgiveness, healing cannot take place. No wonder Jesus told his disciples, "Forgive your brother from your heart" (Matthew 18:35). From-the-heart forgiveness restores relationships and promotes inner healing. Without it, our anger turns inward and can manifest itself both physically and psychologically in insomnia, heart disease, depression, and other ailments.

Anger itself is not wrong. The psalmist said, "In your anger do not sin; when you are on your beds, search your hearts and be silent" (Psalm 4:4). But we just dig ourselves in deeper when we dwell on the cause of our anger, do not acknowledge what we have contributed to the problem, and plot revenge. This is a sure way to keep sleep away.

Whatever the cause of our anger—whether from trivial hurts or serious transgressions—don't let it outlive the day. Don't go to bed angry. If we do, we suffer, our families suffer, and so does everyone else around us.

It may be terribly hard, but choose to forgive others, whether or not they deserve it. Let your anger go. Surrender it to God. Doing so gives closure to the day and ushers in the night with peace.

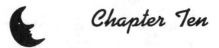 *Chapter Ten*

# The Spiritual Connection

*Finding Rest for the Soul*

When asked what insomniacs want more than anything, most would reply, "A full night's sleep, of course!" But I'm not sure that's exactly true. Our quest for rest asks for more than just one night of sound slumber. Eight consecutive hours of sleep can't erase the effects of weeks or even years of receiving too little rest. We want more than one night. Much more. Most of us are seeking a more *genuine rest*— "Not just the 'good night's sleep' kind of rest that satisfies the body, but an internal rest that bathes the soul in contentment."[1]

If you have worked your way this far through the book, you know by now that I believe all the sleep remedies and prescriptions can go only so far in helping you cope with your insomnia. To truly find rest— real rest of the soul as well as the body—we must move beyond the solutions that look only at physical, psychological, and emotional concerns. We must talk about spiritual truths.

I once passed a church with a sign out front that

read: "Don't count sheep. Talk to the Shepherd." That's an interesting alternative to a time-honored sleep solution, don't you think? While there is nothing wrong with counting farm animals (it can work for people with certain forms of insomnia or for short periods of time), this saying refers to the other dimension of rest which is the focus of this chapter.

## A New Perspective

In the quiet, undistracted darkness of night, I've come to the conclusion that finding my rest in God is more important than just sleeping through the night. If I'm willing, I can use those sleepless hours to become more sensitive to God's presence, more acutely aware of how much I need him. It's impossible to feel totally self-sufficient when my body and mind can't get to sleep despite their overwhelming weariness. I silently unload my fears and frustrations, my nocturnal isolation, and my desperation to God. Although I've believed in him for a long time, I find myself relating to him more authentically and humbly in the middle of the night. When all the day's pretense is peeled away, I can allow myself to be completely honest with him.

Most of us work hard striving to ensure our own sense of security and significance in life. We may look to our own abilities, to other people, or even to society to take care of our needs and affirm us. Yet because we are spiritual beings, as well as physical and psychological beings, we function best when we connect our needs and problems to God's supplies and solutions.

My life was radically changed when I came to believe that God sent Jesus into the world so people could experience a full life, "real and eternal life, more and better life than [we] ever dreamed of" (John 10:10, *The Message*). This new life includes an underlying peace that transcends how well we sleep on any given night. This understanding helped me respond to Jesus' words: "Come to me, all you who are weary and burdened, and I will give you *rest*" (Matthew 11:28, italics mine). Jesus invited the people he lived among long ago to bring their burdens to him, and he offers us the same invitation today.

Doesn't it make beautiful sense that the God who designed our days and nights can help us learn to function our best at *all* times? Whatever our circumstances, true rest comes only when we choose to believe that God is able and willing to take care of us, no matter what, no matter when.

## Learning to Trust

Many of you who are reading these words experience God's closeness in your lives. My intent in this book has been to share something of the sleep process as well as give practical advice and spiritual reminders to add to your artillery for battling sleeplessness.

Others of you may have followed many of the suggestions in this book and perhaps even undergone medical tests, yet you find rest still elusive. If the Bible is true, genuine soul rest will become part of your life only when you enter a relationship with God based on trust. If you have never thought about the need for such a connection, won't you take time now to consider it?

God's plan is to bring people into his family, to a place where they can find rest living within his loving limits. The Bible claims that all human beings are inclined to go their own way instead of God's way.

Some people find this a difficult premise to accept. After all, our culture insists that everyone is basically good. Yet when all illusion is stripped away, we realize how determined we are to serve our own selfish interests—pleasure, self-fulfillment, wealth, and more. If we pursue this path, we find it leads to heartache and inevitable death, rather than the rest we desire. If we follow God's plan through his Son Jesus Christ, we'll find that he gives us everything we need for a life of love and purpose and rest, whether we're awake or asleep.

God is continually calling us to come to him. "The promise of 'arrival' and 'rest' is still there for God's people. . . . And at the end of the journey we'll surely rest with God. So let's keep at it and eventually arrive at the place of rest, not drop out through some sort of disobedience" (Hebrews 4:9-11, *The Message)*. We can choose whether to turn away from him or toward him. When we open our hearts and minds to receive his gifts of freedom and fulfillment, we will find soul rest, and we may find that our bodies will rest better too. How liberating to turn our lives and all our cares over to Jesus Christ and travel with him on the journey to life.[2]

If this is your heart's desire, join me in saying this prayer: "Lord Jesus, I realize that I've been living to please myself and that this isn't the right or best way to live. Thank you for dying on the cross and offering me the gift of eternal life. Please forgive me and lead me on your path to rest, joy, and love. Amen."

## Discovering God's Presence in Prayer

When you think of prayer, what comes to mind? Some people believe that prayer is just wishful thinking or submitting a list of requests to a "higher power." Others consider prayer to be a formal way of addressing God by repeating words designed for that purpose. The following definition comes closer to what I have learned about prayer over the years: *Prayer is two-way communication between God and his people.* That simple.

We can talk with God about anything. Most people of prayer tell God their deepest needs and desires, as well as praise him for who he is. Sleepless nights give us wonderful opportunities to pray for other people in our lives, such as family members, friends, co-workers, and neighbors.

Prayers may be expressed silently or aloud, because God hears our thoughts as well as our words. Therefore, we can pray in the nighttime without disturbing the sleeping members of our households. These quiet hours are also conducive to the "listening" side of prayer, which is often difficult to practice in days filled with noise and interruptions. Sometimes I write out my prayers, because in the act of writing I'm better able to articulate my inner thoughts and feelings. It's also easier to thank God for ways he answered my prayers when I can look back on what I wrote earlier.

Prayer refocuses our thoughts and priorities and helps us turn our anxieties over to God. Through the act of praying (which my friend Del always reminds me is a privilege), we grow closer to God. As we spend time with him and seek his guidance, he takes our lives in new and positive directions.

## Reading the Bible for Encouragement

Someone once shared with me his favorite get-to-sleep strategy. "When I can't sleep," he said, "I just begin reading the book of Leviticus. It works every time!"

I have also found rest by reading the Bible, though not in the same way. A few years ago I began researching what God had to say about nighttime and how people living centuries ago spent their nights. I was impressed by the amount of information and comfort I found in Scripture that spoke directly to the subject. Instead of nodding off, I journaled my discoveries, and a book was born: *Spiritual Nightlights: Meditations for the Middle of the Night.*[3]

The Bible always surprises me with its relevance to whatever situation I find myself in. Its invaluable, timeless inspiration is as true for those of us who experience wakeful nights as it is for people who struggle with other problems. Whenever I read a different translation of the Bible, its familiar words come alive in a fresh way. This might be true for you too, so try reading a newer version or paraphrase of the Bible. As you read, meditate on the words. Transform them into prayers. Begin keeping a journal of what you discover about God and about yourself through the verses you read.

There's a rhythm to life—a time to work and a time to rest, a time to give and a time to receive, a time to act, and a time to simply trust God to work all things out for our good. Even when we can't change our situation or environment to accommodate our need for sleep or anything else, God's power can overrule; he can change things. He wants our bodies to have rest, yes, but even more than that, he wants our souls to find rest in him.

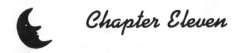 *Chapter Eleven*

# The Family Connection

## *Your Child's Sleep Needs*

"Oh, to be able to sleep like a baby!" Terry sighed wistfully. I started to agree with her, then checked myself. After all, infants usually don't sleep through the night until they are at least three months of age. Some don't accomplish this until their tenth month. That means a lot of lost sleep for their parents, who look for creative ways of surviving that difficult period.

Of course, babies look angelic and carefree as they snooze in their cribs. But anyone who has lived with one knows that the slightest discomfort can ruin their peaceful slumber. In turn, they disturb the peace of whoever is within earshot. No, "sleeping like a baby" is definitely a misnomer.

One reason families exist is to nurture children from their tiniest, most vulnerable stage on through childhood and adolescence until they become mature adults. Parents help fulfill this plan when they provide their offspring with a safe environment, comfort when needed, and the resources needed to meet life's challenges—including sleeplessness.

As parents, we will find it easiest to start establishing sensible sleep habits in our children's lives as early as possible. This chapter offers time-honored suggestions for how to settle a newborn to sleep, then looks at how to aid older children in getting a good night's sleep, even if they have already developed some difficulties. It's never too late to initiate sleep training, but it always comes easier if you start at the beginning.

## Infants and Sleep

Often a person's greatest adjustment to parenthood is getting a newborn to sleep so Mom and Dad can rest, too. Yet overanxious parents may create sleep problems for their babies without realizing it. For example, by always rocking your baby to sleep, you may set yourself up for a repeat performance at every nap and bedtime for months to come. To prevent this, put your infant in her crib while drowsy but not yet asleep. You want her to be aware that she is in her bed before she dozes off completely. In this way she will learn that your arms are not the only secure place to let herself give in to sleep.

Charles Schaefer, Ph.D., director of the Better Sleep Center at Fairleigh Dickinson University in Hackensack, New Jersey, says that it's okay to allow a baby to have a special blanket or toy as a soother. She will soon associate that object with sleep and become less dependent on you for transitioning her into the sleep state.

Babies are erratic sleepers, waking unexpectedly for any number of reasons. Determining the particular cause of each awakening is usually accomplished only by trial and error. Eventually you will come to recognize your infant's differing cries and needs. One wail might mean, "I'm hungry," while another type tells parents, "I need a diaper change." From silent tears to loud bawling, little ones make their needs known. Because discomfort is usually the reason their sleep is disrupted, be sure to check the following:

*Is she too hot or too cold?* Babies don't conserve body heat well, nor can they regulate their own body temperatures by adding or removing blankets or items of clothing. They depend on you for that. Make sure your baby has a warm blanket and perhaps pajamas with feet to keep her warm. Check also for overheating, especially in hot weather. If the back of your baby's neck is damp, she is too warm.

*Does his diaper need to be changed?* Check to see if it is soaked or soiled.

*Is her stomach full of gas?* Gas is painful, causing your baby to waken with a shrill wail. Try burping your baby to make her more comfortable. If this is a chronic problem, see your physician for assistance. Your baby may have colic and need medical attention.

*Is he merely unsettled or wound up?* Try walking him, rocking to soft music, or singing to him. Repetitive movement and rhythmic sounds are comforting to little ones. Again, place him back in the crib just before he falls asleep.

## How Much Sleep Do Children Need?

Just as adults' sleep needs vary from one individual to the next, so do children's. However, knowing approximately how much sleep a child in a certain age group is likely to need can provide a guideline for helping us decide if a child requires more shuteye.

| Age | Sleep needed per 24-hour period |
| --- | --- |
| Newborns | 18 hours, divided into short periods throughout day and night |
| 2-18 months | Nightly sleep block grows longer, daytime sleep into predictable nap times |
| 2 years | 10-13 hours, plus an afternoon nap |
| 3-5 years | 10-12 hours, gradually giving up their nap |
| 6-10 years | 10 hours at least |

To estimate how many hours of sleep your individual child needs, check the chart above and ask yourself these questions:

*How soundly does my child sleep at night?* If he wakes often in the night, he is probably experiencing some sort of sleep disturbance.

*Do her sleep habits seem irregular?* If she has difficulty getting up in the morning, or if she falls asleep in the middle of the day (apart from a scheduled nap time, if she has one), she probably isn't getting enough sleep.

*Does he show signs of irritability, sluggishness, hyperactivity, or difficulty concentrating?* Any one of these may indicate some amount of sleep deprivation. Pay close attention to his moods and behaviors.

*Does she suffer from headaches and other minor physical ailments?* These might also indicate that a child needs more sleep.

*How long does he sleep when allowed to go as long as he likes?* My friend Pat said, "Our pediatrician suggested that during a school vacation we set a consistent bedtime for our daughter, Mandy. We let her sleep in each morning until she woke up on her own.

This helped us figure out how many hours of sleep Mandy really needed."

## Establishing a Bedtime Routine

To cultivate good sleep habits in your children, be faithful in both the timing and rituals of bedtime. The steps of your routine will help ensure that your children receive a good night's sleep.

*1. Plan to put your children to bed at the same time each night and wake them at the same time each morning.* Set the times based on your family's schedules and each child's individual sleep needs, being as consistent as you can. This may vary somewhat over the years, as it did for one family I know. When the father's work hours changed, his family shifted the children's bedtimes so they could spend time with their dad.

*2. Begin helping your children wind down at least one hour before bedtime.* Many children become hyperactive as they grow more tired. Overtired, overexcited children find it difficult to get to sleep. Help them relax by spending between thirty minutes to an hour performing predictable, calming rituals, like brushing teeth and getting into pajamas.

"My wife and I view our children's bedtime as the most critical time of their daily routine," Tim Kimmel writes. "Before Mr. Sandman leans over the edge of their covers to sprinkle sleep dust into their eyes, we like to sprinkle some rest into their souls."[1]

*3. As bedtime draws closer, begin final preparations.* This is when you turn out the light (and perhaps turn on a night-light), say prayers, and give each child a goodnight hug and kiss. Such habits comfort children and give them a sense of security and belonging. Performing these rituals in the same sequence each night communicates order, which further calms a tired child. This regular time also fulfills their need for your undivided attention and builds intimate bonds between you.

"As we watch our children outgrow favorite toys, favorite songs, and favorite pillows," Kimmel says, "we know they must soon outgrow this little bedtime ritual as well. So these special times of reflection and perspective must not be taken lightly. The calmness of spirit passed on to our children must serve them in the darkest hours of their lives."[2]

## Changing Poor Sleep Habits

As I stated earlier, it's never too late to retrain your children in their sleep habits, but it will take determination and perseverance. Do any of the following sound too familiar?

### "I want a drink of water!"
Your child may be really thirsty. Or, perhaps more than a drink, your child may crave some parental attention in the night, or has fears of the dark. Try spending more one-on-one time with her during the day and especially just before bedtime to fill this need. Reassure her that you are nearby; turn on a night-light if needed. Then tell her to go to sleep.

If this request for a drink has become an annoyingly repetitious problem, don't give in to the temptation to fetch the requested water. It won't solve the problem and might create other difficulties, such as the need to go to the bathroom later in the night. Once you have responded to your child's first call and made sure things are okay, leave the room. Depending on her age, the child may cry, get her own water, or just go back to sleep.

### "I'm scared of the dark."

Because you don't want to confuse your child's internal body clock and his sensitivity to nature's cycles of light and darkness, don't make his bedroom too bright at night. He might develop other sleep problems. A night-light should give off enough illumination to do the trick. If that doesn't answer your child's immediate need, turn on a light, then dim it a bit more each night.

### "Can I sleep with you?"

In many cultures around the world, sharing a "family bed" is not unusual. However, in Western cultures, parents consider their bedroom privacy beneficial to their marriage and, therefore, to their family as a whole. It isn't harmful for young children to share their parents' bed—as long as they do not view sexual activities between their mother and father—but crowded conditions often result in poor sleep for everyone in the family. If a child grows accustomed to the family bed, she may have difficulty getting to sleep in other settings she will encounter throughout her life.

If you want to stop a child's dependency on sleeping in your bed (except perhaps to cuddle in the morning or when she is sick), first talk it over with her. Try to discover any underlying reason that compels her to sleep in your bed rather than her own. Then be prepared to escort her back to her bedroom several times a night for up to a month. If the problem persists after that, seek professional help with the situation.

## The Teen Years

School systems in Minnesota have responded to adolescents' difficulties awakening in the morning and excessive daytime sleepiness by delaying the start of the middle-school day until 8:40 A.M. and the high school until 9:40 A.M. They did so because scientific evidence has shown that body clocks, which control waking and sleeping schedules, are slower during the teen years. Research indicates that teenagers often don't become fully awake until 3:00 in the afternoon, just as their school day is ending.

A slower body clock combined with an increase in after-school extracurricular and social activities lead to irregular sleep patterns. An early wake-up time contributes to a growing sleep debt or students' oversleeping on school days. By trying to make up for this lost sleep on weekends, they further disrupt their already-confused internal clocks.

College students often fall victim to insomnia as they leave a structured home life and enter a dormitory or apartment environment. New academic, social, and emotional challenges arise at the same time that they are coping with the need to determine their own sleep-wake schedules. How well they adapt to this change can determine how well they will adjust to a business schedule after graduation.

Sleep deprivation in teens needs to be taken seriously. It can signal depression, drug use, narcolepsy, or a condition called "phase delay insomnia," which may lead to problems at school or work. These conditions can be treated successfully by psychologists, physicians, and/or sleep disorders specialists.

## Sleepwalking

Sleepwalking or *somnambulism* is common in children, especially between the ages of six and twelve, but they usually outgrow the condition. (See the discussion of delayed sleep phase syndrome in chapter 7.) It tends to run in families. Sleepwalking is affected by psychological factors, and it occurs more often in a child who is tense or anxious.

Contrary to popular belief, sleepwalking can be dangerous, especially if the child trips over objects, falls down a flight of stairs, or leaves the safety of home. Therefore, parents should take precautionary measures, such as having the somnambulant child sleep in a first-floor bedroom if possible, and installing door and window locks or even an alarm system to alert the parents if the child gets out of bed in the night.

## Sleep Terrors

*Crash!* A sudden loud noise came from my daughter Taryn's room where I had put her to bed an hour earlier. I found her sitting up in bed in a state of panic. Her eyes were open but unfocused, and she was crying hysterically. Her bedside lamp lay on the floor.

"What happened, honey?" I asked as I tried to take her in my arms. She threw off my attempts to comfort her. She seemed terrified of something I could not see. Whatever it was, it caused her to tremble, sweat, and gasp for breath. She refused to let me hold her, but I stayed with her until she eventually settled down without waking. Oddly, she didn't remember the incident in the morning.

This sort of thing happened several times when Taryn was young. I soon learned that she was experiencing "sleep terrors." They tend to run in families, and, sure enough, I found out my husband had also experienced sleep terrors as a child. They are most common in children between the ages of four and twelve, more often affecting boys than girls, and usually cease by adolescence. They happen more often when the child has a fever or an irregular sleep schedule. On occasion, sleep terrors may involve sleepwalking as well.

If children prone to sleep terrors are disturbed early in the night during their deepest sleep, their brains awaken halfway. It is in this semiconscious state that sleep terrors occur.

Experts advise against forcing your child to wake completely (it's almost impossible anyway). Give verbal reassurance and stay close by until the episode is over. My mother-in-law said that my husband's sleep terrors stopped when she ceased serving him a bedtime snack. If your child has sleep terrors, you might want to give this a try.

## Nightmares

In contrast to sleep terrors, nightmares are frightening dreams that occur in the second half of the night during REM sleep, and they usually wake the sleeper. Children and adults alike suffer from these vivid and terrifying dreams, although they usually diminish with age. Often, nightmares occur in times of stress or after some trauma. Because small children may react strongly to images on television, restrict TV watching for at least one hour prior to bedtime.

If your child experiences a nightmare, let him talk

about it and comfort him. Because nightmares make the dreamer feel helpless, I have found it helpful to pray with my children after a bad dream, drawing on God's power to conquer the nightmare stimulus. Those with long-term recurring nightmares may find they need psychological counseling to resolve the problem.

## Bed-wetting

If your child wets the bed at night, be assured that this problem is relatively common in children, especially up to the age of five. And it may continue as late as the early teen years. Bed-wetting, or enuresis, is more common in boys than girls.

For a child under six years of age, try not to make an issue of bed-wetting. It usually indicates that the bladder's sphincter muscle is slow in maturing. Chances are, he or she will grow out of it. By the age of five, about 85 percent of children have achieved nighttime bladder control. Ninety-nine percent of childhood bed-wetters are continent by the time they finish puberty.

For older children, you will want to check with your family doctor or pediatrician to find out if there is a medical cause for the problem. Besides slow development, bed-wetting may be triggered by a stressful change in the child's life (a new baby's arrival, a family conflict, starting school, etc.). Bed-wetting might also signal a urinary tract infection, kidney disorder, hormonal upset, a lag in nerve connections to the bladder, or other physical problem. Consult your child's physician if pain is present. Your child's doctor may also prescribe another appropriate medication such as imipramine.

Here are some steps you can take on your own to help correct a child's bed-wetting.

❧ Never punish your child or make him feel ashamed. Bed-wetting is an involuntary act, and parental anger can damage a child's self-esteem. However, if he is old enough, have him take responsibility for changing and washing his bedding. This has been shown to actually improve a child's self-worth.

❧ Limit your child's fluid intake from late afternoon on, and make sure he empties his bladder just before bed.

❧ Some experts advise bladder-stretching exercises to help the body accommodate a greater amount of liquid. To do this, have your child drink a large amount of fluid early in the day and delay going to the bathroom to gain more bladder control.

❧ Build the child's sphincter muscle strength by having him start and stop his urine flow midstream when he goes to the bathroom during the day.

❧ You may want to invest in a bell-and-pad self-training method, in which a bell wakens the sleeper whenever urine hits the rubber pad on which he is lying.

❧ Try setting an alarm to awaken the sleeping child every two hours throughout the night, alerting the child to his need to urinate.

❧ Ask your physician about the nasal spray DDAVP (desmopressin acetate). This is an artificial version of a normal body hormone that slows nightly urine production. It is especially effective when used with an alarm that is activated by the first few drops of urine.

   ❧ Above all, be supportive and encourage your child to talk openly with you about his concerns. Be matter-of-fact, adopt a positive attitude, and work together toward the goal of a dry night's sleep.

Insomnia in children should be taken seriously, because it could signal the presence of childhood-onset (or primary) insomnia—the lifelong inability to obtain adequate sleep. Scientists believe this organic problem may be caused by a chemical imbalance or nervous system dysfunction involved with the sleep process. People with this problem are highly sensitive to noise, light, and any type of stimulant.

If you or your child has struggled with sleep for as long as you can remember, be sure to follow sleep-hygiene rules carefully, such as getting enough exercise, learning to manage stress, staying away from caffeine, reducing noise and light in your bedroom, and so on. Sleeping pills are usually ineffective in treating childhood-onset insomnia, but low dosages of antidepressants often help by changing the biochemical balance in the brain. Check with your doctor for help in extreme cases.

You can start your child on a lifelong pattern of good sleep practices by beginning in infancy. But remember: no matter what age, it's never too late to start.

# Chapter Twelve

# The Marriage Connection

*Supporting Your Sleepless Spouse*

"I've never had trouble sleeping in my life. I'm out the minute my head hits the pillow. I don't understand why my wife can't sleep. What's wrong with her?"

"My husband snores so loudly, he wakes himself up. Sometimes it sounds like he stops breathing. I'm worried about him."

"My wife is such a light sleeper. If I so much as roll over, she wakes up. I feel badly about it."

Insomnia can bring some interesting challenges to a marriage. We make vows to honor each other "for better or for worse," but maybe a promise to love "in waking and in sleeping" should be added.

When your spouse suffers from sleeplessness, you may feel frustrated by your inability to "fix" the problem. Your spouse's tossing and turning disrupts not only his or her own sleep but often yours as well. You can't ignore the impact on your marriage when your partner has difficulty sleeping. Besides nighttime wakefulness, insomnia's effects spill over into the next day as moodiness, irritability, and difficulty coping with stress.

To become more compatible in your sleep habits, it's important to learn about this condition. You *can* help each other through those wakeful nights.

## Affirm Your Loved One

Insomnia is an affliction that threatens its victim's self-esteem. Because of insomnia's repercussions, you as a spouse will find it useful to learn more about it, just as you would if your marriage partner were diagnosed with a life-threatening illness. By doing so, you affirm the serious nature of the struggle and strengthen your partner's self-esteem. As you become more informed, you also will be better equipped to help your life partner deal with the problem.

Begin by trying to discover why your spouse is up at night.

*Is your spouse coping with loss (a death, children leaving home, a broken friendship, etc.)?* When Joan's mother died, she found herself wandering through the house at night, thinking over the past, pondering the future.

After Tom's daughter left for college, he struggled with sleep, wondering if he had been a good father and missing her presence. The house seemed so empty now.

Joan's husband and Tom's wife learned that listening is one of the most valuable tools available to help someone who is grieving. Their spouses—and yours—often need for you to walk through the dark valley with them and encourage them along the way. That may be all the help they need to move back into the groove of healthy sleep patterns.

*Does your spouse suffer from a medical condition that affects sleep?* After numerous medical tests,

Pamela was diagnosed with fibromyalgia. She soon learned that a common symptom of the disease is insomnia. Many other illnesses and some of the medications used to treat these conditions also disrupt sound sleep. When the physical problem is treated or a medication changed, the patient will usually return to former sleep patterns.

*Is your spouse experiencing stress?* When Jim prepares for important business meetings, his tension level climbs as high as it did before he awaited surgery five years ago. A few days preceding each presentation, he lies awake for hours. Stress, whether short- or long-term, builds throughout the day and keeps sleep away at night.

Karen found that each stage of life presented her with new responsibilities. Because she took her obligations seriously, she spent many nights tossing and turning over things her husband considered mundane. When he recognized her need to talk over her concerns with him and receive his support, her sleep habits began to improve.

*Are your spouse's work or sleep patterns irregular?* Recognize that a constantly changing internal clock usually impairs a good night's sleep. Dan worked at a high-stress job and needed a good night's sleep. His wife, Wendy, was a pediatrician, often on-call at night. She went to bed when her husband did, but each time the telephone summoned her, Dan would awaken and be unable to return to sleep. After a call, Wendy would leave for the hospital or deal with the problem over the phone. She would return to bed, unless she was too wound up to sleep. Then she would read or watch television, keeping herself occupied until she was sleepy again. Dan had trouble sleeping with a light on and activity in the same room.

Eventually, they reached a compromise. When Wendy was on-call, Dan slept in the guest room. When Wendy was not on-call, they resumed their normal sleep habits.

*Is your spouse struggling with fear?* Sharon had sleeping problems for several years. Her husband, Pete, traveled for his company and was often gone overnight. Acting on a hunch, Pete installed a security system in their home and bought Sharon a puppy for her birthday. These steps helped her feel safer while Pete was away. Feeling more secure at night, her insomnia disappeared almost immediately.

*Do you have habits that disturb your spouse's ability to rest?* When someone struggles with not sleeping, different preferences or annoying habits can be more upsetting than they are in the light of day. John and Barb have been married eleven years and still disagree about the purpose of a snooze alarm. John likes the luxury of setting the alarm early and hitting the snooze button a few times. Barb, who often barely gets to sleep before the alarm rings, prefers that the alarm go off only once, when it is time to get up.

Nighttime's distraction-free hours give people more time to think and, for some, that's time to worry and fret. Help your spouse keep his or her concerns in proper perspective. Become your spouse's mirror, reflecting reality and correcting distorted perspectives.

Above all, refrain from comparing your spouse to yourself or to others. When people experience guilt over their inability to sleep, unfair comparisons worsen the problem. A person's sleep practices are an individual matter. Acknowledge the differences and avoid arguing about them. Your goal—one that will benefit both of you—is to help your spouse get a good night's rest and to help him or her cope when that does not happen.

## Examine Your Lifestyle

Take the initiative to investigate how your lifestyle and your "sleep hygiene" as a couple contribute to your spouse's wakefulness. Then consider these ways you could bring about change.

*1. Give your spouse time to wind down before bedtime.* Perhaps you could put the children to bed more often, giving her time to read, take a bath, or do whatever she finds most relaxing. A couple friends of mine put on soft music each evening to quiet their minds and prepare their bodies for rest.

*2. Encourage your spouse to exercise.* Suggest taking an early evening walk together, or encourage him to start a regular exercise routine. This helps reduce stress and is a healthy way to tire the body.

*3. Offer to give your partner a backrub or massage.* If you feel awkward about this or don't know how, you could take a class together or seek advice from a massage therapist. There are many books on the subject.

*4. Arrange a good time to make love.* For many people, sexual relations bring sleep more quickly, but for some it works in just the opposite way. If sexual activity keeps your spouse awake long afterwards, change the time when you make love. Be sensitive to your spouse's response and adjust accordingly.

*5. Move up your dinnertime, if possible.* Overeating or eating too close to bedtime increases the chance that the digestive process will interfere with sleep. Eating a lighter meal earlier in the evening often helps a person get to sleep more quickly.

For other specific problems, refer to the chapters in this book that address the particular issues your loved one struggles with.

## The Importance of Communication

Suppressed emotions keep many people awake. If you believe this is a problem for your spouse, offer opportunities to verbalize thoughts and feelings. Communicating in the following ways may lead to better sleeping and can only enhance your marriage.

*Communicate with each other.* Ask questions, take your time, and really listen to the answers. Even if you don't find the solution for sleepless nights, you will grow closer and improve your relationship as you talk together and build trust.

*Communicate with a counselor.* If your problems are too overwhelming to handle alone, you may want to discuss them in the presence of a trusted professional counselor or pastor. This will also assist those couples for whom communication upsets rather than soothes. Everyone finds marriage a difficult challenge at times, and counseling can help you build a stronger, happier marriage.

*Communicate with God.* Christian marriage is often symbolized as a triangle. God is at the peak, the husband and wife are at the two lower corners, and lines connect each to the other. When God is the head of a marriage, the human participants are held together through the storms of life by his love. You will find that nothing is outside the reach of your heavenly Father's loving arms.

For deep communication on a spiritual level, spend time praying together. Jesus said, "When two of you get together on anything at all on earth and make a prayer of it, my Father in heaven goes into action.

And when two or three of you are together because of me, you can be sure that I'll be there" (Matthew 18:19, *The Message*). Later, the apostle James spoke these words: "Make this your common practice: Confess your sins to each other and pray for each other so that you can live together whole and healed" (James 5:16, *The Message*). Praying and listening to God together is a practice that draws on divine power and brings you closer in spirit.

## Be Considerate

Gayle told me that sometimes, as she climbs into bed, her husband says, "I hope you can get to sleep quickly tonight."

"I feel such pressure when he says that!" she told me. "He's trying to encourage me, but instead my body stiffens and I can't get to sleep."

To give your spouse the support he or she needs, determine what they find relaxing and what makes them more tense. Respond lovingly. Here are some suggestions that will help:

- ❧ Be flexible and creative when reconciling your differing sleep schedules. If one marriage partner is a "lark" and the other an "owl," work together to find a sleep routine you can both live with.

- ❧ Negotiate the use of the "snooze button" on your alarm clock. Just as a lights-out preference can sabotage an entire night's sleep, so alarm-clock feuds can spoil the first few hours of the morning.

- ❧ Get help for any of your own sleep habits (snoring, for example) that disturb your spouse's rest. There are many remedies for these on the market, so consult your physician for guidance.

   &#8476; If your partner needs a quiet environment in which to sleep, give the gift of silence. Don't insist on watching TV in bed while your spouse is trying to doze off. (In fact, watching TV in bed is never a good idea. Your bed should be reserved for sleeping or making love.)

   &#8476; Find a "middle ground" for sleeping positions that are comfortable for you both. This may involve changing the size of your bed or talking about personal space issues. Your needs may change over time. Couples who have shared the same bed over many years grow accustomed to their partners' movements, and consequently their sleep is disturbed less often. In addition, simply switching to a larger bed often solves some of these problems.

   &#8476; In extreme cases, consider sleeping separate. A study conducted by Dr. Jim Horne found that when one partner moves, the other usually moves within the next thirty seconds. While most participants felt they slept better with their partner at their side, the study revealed that these same individuals actually experienced fewer interruptions when they slept in a bed by themselves.

Sleeping in separate beds or even separate bedrooms is a last resort for incompatible bed partners. This need not diminish the marriage. As long as couples have a loving relationship and continue their marital relations, it doesn't matter whether or not they actually spend the entire night in the same bed or even the same room. And the courtesy and love shown in wanting to enhance the other's sleep may well add to the quality of your relationship.

## Take Action

If the above suggestions prove ineffective, try some of these ideas for follow-up. By being proactive you will be showing tremendous support for your spouse in his or her struggle with insomnia.

Always be on the lookout for new ideas, books, or articles to encourage your spouse on the journey toward rest. Check the self-help section on the subject of insomnia at your local bookstore and library. Ask for those resources that are most frequently used or requested. Find help online in one of the numerous sleep-related sites on the Internet. See appendix B for websites.

Locate an insomnia support group in your community and encourage your spouse to join, if they have not already done so. In this sympathetic atmosphere, other sufferers share their struggles, suggest sleep aids they have found successful, and work together toward a common goal.

Accompany your spouse when he or she consults a physician or sleep specialist. This will help you better understand your partner's needs. One couple I know always tries to go with each other to medical appointments because they find they remember data and suggestions better when both are present. They are also more able to help each other follow doctors' recommendations.

If you observe symptoms of a sleep disorder in your mate, take action. Partners are the natural observers of sleep-disorder symptoms. Your watchfulness can lead to quicker diagnosis and treatment. For example, when Joyce noticed that her husband, Tim, seemed to stop breathing at times in the night, she recognized it as a symptom of sleep apnea, a serious but treatable condition. They discussed it with his physician, who sent him to a sleep specialist. After a night in a sleep lab, Tim was diagnosed with apnea and helpful treatment began.

## Be Patient

As you and your spouse live through nights together, remember that just as his or her sleeplessness developed over time, it will take time to overcome. Don't expect instant solutions or a quick fix. To do so creates greater stress, perhaps making the problem worse. Spouses who are secure in their partners' love, when encouraged by patient support, will make speedier progress toward more restful nights.

I close this chapter with a true story that will encourage you to hang in there with your sleepless spouse. Mary suffered from insomnia the entire first year and a half of her marriage. Already a light sleeper, the changes and adjustments of marriage had turned her into a serious insomniac.

Her anxiety level would rise each evening as bedtime approached and she became fearful that she wouldn't be able to sleep. Once in bed, worries would crowd her mind. She'd get up, watch movies, cry, write angry letters to God, cry some more, and finally fall asleep on the couch.

"What helped me the most," Mary told me, "was my husband's support and love. He couldn't understand it—he slept through anything. But he didn't judge me, didn't get angry. He just held me when I was at my wit's end and supported me and encouraged me to pursue help."

But her insomnia was wreaking emotional and physical havoc on both of them. Her husband began sleeping more lightly, afraid to even turn over or move because he might wake her up. And everybody stayed away from her during the day due to her crabby moods. Things were pretty desperate.

Mary finally went to a psychiatrist who prescribed some light nonaddictive sleeping pills. It turned out to be the short-term solution she needed to get back into a regular rhythm of sleep.

"I'm learning better how to lay aside my worries and relax. I wear earplugs to block out noises that bother me. And now I can hardly sleep when my husband isn't there beside me. I call that a miracle!"

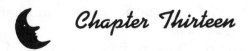 *Chapter Thirteen*

# The Professional Connection

*Seeking the Help You Need*

"SLEEP SALE!" proclaimed the newspaper advertisement. What? Sleep for sale? I was captivated. Of course, the store's newspaper ad only promoted its sale of beds and mattresses, but, wrestling with insomnia, I sure wished I *could* buy sleep. If a company could guarantee its customers a good night's rest without side effects, eager customers would surely overwhelm it with business.

If you have worked your way through this book, tried the suggestions, and still cannot achieve a full night of sound sleep, it is probably time to seek professional advice—if you haven't already done so.

## Your Family Physician

Because untreated sleep problems can become chronic and more difficult to resolve, discuss your sleepless nights with your primary care physician. The aware doctor will take your complaints seriously, review your medical history, and perform a physical examination and laboratory tests. They may suggest further adjustments in your attitude or daily habits or prescribe a medication to help your sleep pattern become normal again.

Your physician also may refer you to a specialist in another field. For example, psychologists and psychiatrists help their patients cope with anxiety, stress, depression, and other psychological troubles that contribute to sleeplessness. Pulmonary specialists might have alternative treatments for physical causes such as sleep apnea. Neurologists may clarify the identification of such nervous-system conditions as restless legs syndrome.

## Sleep Specialist

If finding a solution to your insomnia proves elusive and you still do not see progress in the amount or quality of your sleep, consult a sleep specialist. This is often the most efficient means of diagnosing sleep problems. A recent study by Peter Hauri, director of Mayo Clinic's Insomnia Research and Treatment Program, found that a single appointment with a sleep specialist, combined with follow-up calls by telephone, eased chronic sleeplessness for 75 percent of the patients in the study.[1] Ask your doctor for a referral or consult one of the sleep organizations in appendix B.

## Inside the Sleep Lab

If your problem requires a sleeping evaluation, you need not dread it. Sleep centers accommodate patients in a friendly, professional environment, one that emphasizes their patients' comfort and well-being.

Currently, more than two thousand sleep centers exist in the United States. They are found in most major cities, and many are accredited by the American Sleep Disorders Association. At these centers many patients are helped by personal consultation and treatment and do not always need to stay a night (or day) in a sleep lab.

Consider Pete's sleep lab experience. Pete had gone to his family doctor, complaining of daytime drowsiness. He believed he wasn't getting enough sleep at night. In addition, his wife had described his snoring as loud, with frequent interruptions in breathing followed by gasps for air. His doctor sent him to a sleep specialist, who decided to test for obstructive sleep apnea.

At 7:00 P.M. Pete walked into the sleep center. He was apprehensive. Although he usually avoided hospitals altogether, he was here to spend the night. And if that was not bad enough, he also had to allow strangers to watch him sleep!

As Pete registered at the admissions desk, a young woman with a friendly smile greeted him. "Hi, my name is Kelly. I'm a technician in the sleep lab," she said, leading the way to the elevator. "Have you ever been to a sleep center before?"

"No. But my doctor wanted to check some things out. I'm not really sure what to expect."

"Not to worry," Kelly said cheerfully, as they boarded the elevator. "It's pretty easy." When the elevator stopped, they walked down a long hall, then through a set of double doors marked: "Quiet please. Patients sleeping." They entered another hallway.

"Over here is our control room." Kelly pointed to a small room nearby. "Let's go in, and you can see what I'll be doing while you sleep." They entered a room where several computers and monitors were arranged on long counters. "Can I get you a soda or something else to drink?" she offered.

"No, thanks," Pete said. "Caffeine keeps me awake."

Kelly nodded. "You're right; it can. But we don't have any caffeinated beverages in the sleep lab—just juices and caffeine-free soda."

"Well, maybe later," Pete said, as his eyes traveled around the room. Each television monitor displayed a room with an empty bed.

"You'll be in this one," Kelly said, pointing to the second screen from the left. "I'll be right across the hall in case you need anything. Let's go see your room."

Pete's "room" was simply but comfortably furnished with a double bed, nightstand, TV, and chair. A door to the left led to a private bathroom.

"When you're ready for bed," Kelly said, "just press this buzzer, and I'll bring you a video that shows exactly what to expect while you're here. By the way, the camera only shows the bed, so when you're in the bathroom or away from the bed, you do have *some* privacy." Kelly left Pete to put on his pajamas.

Pete picked up the duffel bag he had brought with him, changed into shorts and a T-shirt, then pressed the buzzer. Kelly returned and inserted a videotape into the VCR.

The twenty-minute video alleviated some of Pete's concerns about the night ahead. He hadn't expected to be hooked up to so many electrodes, but apparently the process wouldn't be painful.

When the tape ended, Kelly returned, and she began attaching small sensors to Pete's head, chest, and feet with a glue-like substance and tape, describing what she was doing as she went along. "Would you like me to take a picture of you when we get you hooked up? I'll bet your kids would get a kick out of it."

Pete chuckled. "Sure, go ahead."

Kelly continued explaining throughout the connection procedure. "We need to chart the stages of sleep you go through and record the level of oxygen in your blood during the night, your heart rate, eye movements, breathing, leg movements, etc. In case you snore, we're ready to record it—that's what this tiny microphone is for. Now, is anything uncomfortable?"

"Well, nothing hurts, if that's what you mean." Pete looked at his reflection in the mirror. "Do people actually sleep with all of these wires attached?"

Kelly nodded. "You'd be surprised. We can usually get enough information even if patients sleep only a few hours. Now I'll dim the lights, and you can watch TV for awhile. I'll be back later. Just buzz me if you need anything."

She left the room, and Pete settled back on the bed to watch the news. He was surprised a little while later to find that he had dozed off. When he woke up, he pressed the buzzer. Kelly returned to turn off the lights and the television, and Pete slipped under the covers for the night. As he slept, small sensors recorded his brain waves, the airflow from his nose and mouth, his blood oxygen level, respiration, the muscle tone in his face, and the movements of his arms and legs.

## Procedures and Costs

Typically, the day after a patient spends the night at a sleep lab, a polysomnologist reviews the data gathered by the nighttime technician. He makes three or four passes over the data, scores it, and analyzes patterns to prepare an in-depth report for the physician who ordered the study. The several pages of records include both technical notes and a visual summary. The physician then studies the data and diagnoses any existing sleep disorder from a criteria bank of more than eighty disorders established by the American Sleep Disorders Association.[2] The next step of patient care involves treatment, then follow-up.

Besides the type of study Pete underwent, some patients have a "split night study," in which part of the night is spent with a continuous positive airwave pressure (CPAP) mask in place and the other part without it, to compare results and adjust the pressure. Other people have daytime testing, which measures the level of sleepiness throughout the day, so the physician can diagnose or rule out narcolepsy.

A sleep clinic evaluation is expensive—between $200 and $300 for the consultation and about $1,500 for an overnight sleep study. The cost is often covered by insurance, but even if it isn't, it could prove worth the time and money spent to find relief for sleep problems. Another advantage to such sleep analysis is that it can shorten the hospital stays of some patients by correcting any breathing problems that interfere with recovery. With more efficient breathing, patients recover faster from their primary illness.

More than two thousand sleep centers are ASDA-accredited to meet minimum standards. While this is one measure of a center's quality of diagnostics, it is not the only industry standard. A reliable method of determining if you will receive quality care at your local sleep center is to make sure your physician and the recording technologists are credentialed, which

means they have passed a series of professional quali-
fying examinations in their fields.

## Conclusion: Bring on the Night!

When insomnia intrudes into your nights and pushes
your body's natural rhythm out of sync, rest assured
that you are not alone and that you are not helpless.
Insomnia is not an incurable problem! The study of
sleep has made such significant progress that most
people can find a solution for their sleeplessness.

I hope the information offered here will encourage
you to delve into the causes of your sleeplessness and
to take action. My own sleep has improved considerably since I set out to conquer insomnia in my life.
Now when I lie awake (yes, it still happens occasionally), I can usually determine the reason why, recognize the options I have in coping with my wakefulness,
and choose my response accordingly.

So begin the journey. Don't let the fear of insomnia
stop you from finding help and making the changes
you need to make on your way to more sleep-filled
nights.

# Appendix A:
# What You Should Know about
# Medications and Health Remedies

From pain relievers and cough syrups to headache remedies and antacids, pharmacy shelves offer multiple medicines for our maladies. And when over-the-counter drugs don't alleviate what ails us, we turn to physicians to prescribe something for our complaints.

We are looking for relief, of course. Yet many of the medications that ease pain can also disrupt our sleep patterns in significant ways. Reading through this information on current medications and remedies will prove useful in your search for better sleep.

## Medications and Sleep

To discover if your medications are keeping you awake at night, make a list of your prescriptions and over-the-counter medicines. Then check the pharmaceutical instructions for drug side effects. Try to recall what changes of medication were made about the time your sleep problem began.

Discuss this information with your physician. If a new drug is at fault, your doctor may alter your dosage or recommend that you adjust the time of day you take it, so it will have the desired effect and also allow you to get a good night's rest. Or your physician may prescribe a similar medication that will not interfere with your sleep.

Here is a list of drugs that claim insomnia as a potential side effect:[1]

❧ Certain antidepressants
❧ Drugs with amphetamine, such as prescription diet pills
❧ Some drugs that control high blood pressure

- ❧ Some birth control pills (although this is rare)
- ❧ Bronchodilating drugs (for breathing problems) that contain ephedrine, aminophylline, or norepinephrine
- ❧ Medications containing caffeine
- ❧ Sleeping pills and tranquilizers (Insomnia may result from withdrawal on the nights you don't use them.)
- ❧ Steroid preparations
- ❧ Some cancer chemotherapeutic agents
- ❧ Adrenocorticotropic hormone (ACTH)
- ❧ Dopamine
- ❧ Some beta blockers prescribed for hypertension
- ❧ Diuretics (which cause frequent nocturnal urination, thus interfering with sleep)
- ❧ Some thyroid preparations, especially if the dose is not exactly right
- ❧ Appetite suppressants
- ❧ Some cold remedies

## Sleeping Pills

Sleep medications and tranquilizers, once distributed widely, are now being prescribed more selectively. While they do not cure insomnia, they can be an effective weapon against sleeplessness if used for a short time—just until sleep is regulated. However, for insomnia caused by disorders that involve difficulty breathing, they may make the problem even worse. Therefore, it is important to have your insomnia properly diagnosed.

Whether prescribed or purchased over the counter, sleeping pills are not meant to be used on a long-term basis for several reasons. First, drug-induced sleep does not have as high a quality as natural sleep. Sleeping pills may increase the total length of sleep time, but they decrease a person's amount of deep sleep. Second, the pills may work at first, but our bodies eventually build up a tolerance to them. To continue receiving benefits from them, we often have to raise the dose. In addition, such side effects as impaired memory and elevated blood pressure may occur.

Sleep medications help most when treating jet lag, periodic flare-ups of insomnia, or occasional times of stress when sleep eludes us.

Since sleeping pills are most effective for a limited time—a few weeks up to a couple months—why do so many people take them on a long-term basis? First, when stopped abruptly after a long period of use, the user's insomnia may be worse than before he or she started taking the pills. This "rebound insomnia" may continue for several weeks. Second, sleeping medications are psychologically addicting. Even after they lose their effectiveness, some people tend to keep taking them, believing they cannot get to sleep without medicinal help.

*The New England Journal of Medicine* recommends five basic principles to guide the use of medications for chronic insomnia:[2]

1. Use the lowest effective dose.
2. Take sleeping pills intermittently (two to four times weekly).
3. Doctors: prescribe for short-term use (no more than three to four weeks).
4. Withdraw the medication gradually.
5. Watch for rebound insomnia.

Today's most frequently prescribed sleeping pills are the benzodiazepines. If used daily for several months, they can be habit-forming, but they are considered safe if used intermittently. Long-acting medications (e.g., Dalmane) work best for people who struggle with anxiety during the day; short-acting drugs (e.g., Restoril or Halcion) are better for people who are tired in the day and wide-awake at night.[3]

Antidepressants—especially the serotonin-based medications—are sometimes used in low doses to alleviate the sleep disturbances that accompany depression. Some researchers believe that the use of an appropriate antidepressant medication not only prevents major depression but also diminishes the burden of chronic insomnia.[4]

Over-the-counter sleep medications usually contain an antihistamine as a principal ingredient. Unfortunately, their sedative effects can linger into the next day. And our bodies build up a resistance to them. Occasional use is effective if your sleep difficulty occurs just once in a while.

## Herbal Alternatives

Before turning to a pharmacological approach to your insomnia, you may want to experiment with natural remedies. These include lifestyle changes as well as vitamins, herbs, and minerals.

To investigate herbs as an option, first visit your local health food store and ask how to take them. Overdosing, or taking herbs in wrong combinations, can also cause unwanted side effects. Always begin with a low dosage and increase it as necessary.

Herbal food supplements and products to help consumers sleep abound in health food stores. Their manufacturers use scientific discoveries in sleep physiology and nutrient connections along with herbal tradition to develop formulas that allegedly alleviate insomnia. Some products you might find on the store shelves include the following.

## Chamomile
Sipping a cup of chamomile tea is a widely recognized pre-bedtime soother, calming both the mind and the digestive system and making sleep come more quickly. Pleasant-tasting and without side effects, this tea has a long tradition as a natural sleep aid. It is safe enough for children's use.

## Lemon balm
This member of the mint family comes from Europe and is often used for treating herpes sores, nervous hearts or stomachs, and insomnia. To prepare lemon balm *(Melissa officinalis)* tea, add two teaspoonful of the ground leaves to a cup of steaming hot water. Sweeten with a little honey, if desired. Drink a cup after your evening meal and another just before bed.

## Passionflower
The passionflower vine, common in the southeastern United States, is useful in treating symptoms of nervous anxiety or an overactive mind. European medical practitioners advise the use of passionflower for its mild depressive effect on the central nervous system, and they maintain that it is safe. Passionflower is most available in the United States in the form of capsules and tinctures. Some advise combining this product with chamomile tea for use just before going to bed.

## Valerian extract
The herb valerian *(valeriana officinalis)* ranks high on the list of natural sleep aids because of its effectiveness. It has long been

recognized for its qualities as a mild sedative and spasm reducer, as well as its ability to increase coronary blood flow. In a recent Swiss study, researchers found that valerian helped 128 troubled insomniacs drop off to sleep faster and sleep longer than without it.[5]

Valerian also does not seem to have aftereffects the following morning. So far its only drawback is that some individuals experience a stimulant effect or develop headaches from its use. If desired as a sleep aid, try taking two to three grams of the herb after dinner and another dose one hour before bedtime. It is available as capsules or in liquid drops, which are added to water. Valerian may also be made into tea, but many find its odor and taste in this form unpleasant.

## Vitamins and Minerals

### Calcium

One of the most plentiful minerals in the human body, calcium works in conjunction with magnesium to facilitate neuromuscular function. Calcium and magnesium working together relax the nerves and muscles. They also have a sedative effect on brain cells. If your body is deficient in either of these minerals, your brain will be more sensitive to noise, light, odor, touch, etc., which impair your ability to fall asleep.

To ensure that your body gets enough calcium, include dairy products (milk, cheese, yogurt, etc.) in your diet. If this is not possible, eat more spinach, broccoli, sardines, salmon, and/or tofu. For those who prefer to take calcium supplements, choose those made with calcium citrate, because other forms may interfere with iron absorption or cause kidney stones. If you choose calcium carbonate, take it with meals to help its absorption. The recommended amount of calcium per day is about 1,000 milligrams through a combination of diet and supplements (1,500 milligrams for post-menopausal women).

### Vitamin B

If stress and anxiety are primary reasons for your lack of sleep, give the B-complex vitamins a try. B vitamins help calm the nervous system. Take them either in tablet form as a food supplement, or add more whole-wheat bread, cereal, brown rice, nuts, seeds, and green vegetables to your diet.

**Vitamin E**

Recent studies show that *natural* vitamin E has improved the symptoms of restless legs syndrome and nocturnal leg cramps, both of which contribute to insomnia. As few as 200 units of vitamin E helped the surveyed patients find relief from these conditions.

To be sure you're buying natural E, look for the letter "d" in front of the word "tocopherol." (The synthetic form has the letters "dl.")[6]

## Other Non-Drug Therapies

### Tryptophan

This essential amino acid is found in many foods, and it links the brain chemical serotonin to the sleep process. Because our bodies naturally change tryptophan into serotonin, researchers have studied pure tryptophan as a natural sleep inducer. When studies showed that three to five grams of tryptophan, when manufactured in tablet form, helped some people fall asleep more quickly, many people began to use tryptophan tablets for relaxation and sleep.

However, in the late 1980s, more than 1,500 cases of a painful and sometimes fatal disease called eosinophilia-myalgia were linked to an impurity in the tryptophan produced by the Japanese company Showa Denko. During the search for the cause of the disease, all tryptophan tablets were recalled. Costs of product liability and impurity-free production have blocked its return to the market. You can boost the amount of tryptophan in your diet naturally simply by eating a variety of foods such as milk, meat, fish, poulty, beans, cheese, and green leafy vegetables.

### GHB (Gamma hydroxybutyrate)

GHB is in the process of finding its place in sleep medicine. Found in every cell of the human body, GHB was synthesized thirty years ago. It is so powerful and works so quickly, "you're told to go to bed first and *then* take it," says Barry Rosloff, a pharmacologist for the Food and Drug Administration. This compound was sold illegally in the late 1980s and early 1990s, but the Justice Department cracked down on its sale because of reports of overdoses, some of which caused comas.

However, sleep researcher Martin Scharf, at the Tri-State Sleep Disorders Center in Cincinnati, demonstrated the effectiveness of using GHB in treating narcoleptics. GHB allowed them to sleep for longer periods at night, after which they were able to function far better the next day. Currently the substance is being studied for possible approval by the FDA. Researchers believe its benefits might include helping older adults sleep deeper and longer.

### Melatonin

A hormone naturally produced in our body's pineal gland, melatonin is the newest "wonder drug," used as a supplement specifically to induce sleep and overcome jet lag. It appears to keep our internal clocks in sync with the day-night cycles of our environment by informing the brain that darkness has fallen and it's time to rest.

Studies of melatonin have so far yielded inconsistent results. Although it appears to be effective in treating jet lag, researchers find no consensus on its ability to treat insomnia. In fact, it actually seems to reduce the amount of deep sleep by about 40 percent. Researchers also disagree on melatonin's safety when used on a long-term basis, although it has been deemed safe for short-term use. Melatonin is sold in health food stores and pharmacies. See pages 90 and 93 for further discussion.

## Illegal Drugs and Sleep

Wakefulness is one consequence of using illegal drugs such as amphetamines, marijuana, heroin, or cocaine. Reasons for this vary, due to the varying characteristics of the drug. Amphetamines are stimulants. Heroin interferes with breathing and frequently causes the sleeper to return from deeper stages of sleep to the lightest stage. If a young person suddenly exhibits sleeplessness, parents should be alert to possible drug abuse.

# Appendix B:
# Organizations and Web Sites

## Organizations

American Sleep Apnea Association
2025 Pennsylvania Avenue NW
Suite 905
Washington, DC 20006
(202) 293-3650
http://www.nicom.com

American Sleep Disorders Association
1610 14th Street NW, Suite 300
Rochester, MN 55901
http://www.asda.org

Better Sleep Council
333 Commerce Street
Alexandria, VA 22314
(703) 683-8371

Narcolepsy Network
P.O. Box 42460
Cincinnati, OH 45242
(513) 891-3522
E-mail: narnet@aol.com
http://www.websciences.org/narnet

National Institutes of Health
National Center for Sleep Disorders Research
Two Rockledge Centre
Suite 7024
6701 Rockledge Dr. MSC 7920
Bethesda, MD 20892-7920

National Sleep Foundation
729 Fifteenth St. NW
Washington, DC 20005
(202) 347-3471
E-mail: natsleep@erols.com
http://www.sleepfoundation.org

Restless Legs Syndrome (RLS) Foundation
4410 19th Street NW, Suite 201
Rochester, MN 55901
http://www.rls.org

Sleep Disorders Dental Society
11676 Perry Highway Building #1
Suite 1204
Wexford, PA 15090
(412) 935-0836

Sleep/Wake Disorders Canada
3089 Bathurst Street
Suite 304
Toronto, Ontario M6A 2A4
CANADA
(416) 787-5374

Shuteye, a service of the Searle Corporation
P.O. Box 14687
Baltimore, MD 21298-9092
1-800-SHUTEYE for a free sleep kit and brochures

## Web Sites

### Sleep Home Page
http://www.bisleep.medsch.ucla.edu
The Brain Information Service presents research and
treatment of sleep and sleep-related disorders.

**Bibliosleep**

http://www.websciences.org/bibliosleep

Bibliographic references to sleep and sleep-related professional publications from 1994 to the present, with earlier years being added.

**The Shuteye News**

http://www.shuteye.com

The Searle Corporation's online newsletter.

**The Sleep Medicine Home Page**

http://www.cloud9.net/thorpy

Sponsored by the Montefiore Hospital Sleep Disorder Center in New York, this site lists resources on sleep, discussion groups, foundations related to sleep, sleep disorders centers, and other sleep-related information.

**SleepNet**

http://www.sleepnet.com

Sponsored by the Stanford School of Sleep Medicine, this site links sleep information in the Internet about support groups, sleep disorders, treatments, and sleep disorders centers.

# Endnotes

**Introduction**

1. These figures were derived from a projection to the total adult American population (U.S. Census Bureau, March 1997: 197, 497,000) of the finding that 67 percent of respondents reported a sleep symptom. This information was graciously supplied by the National Sleep Foundation, 729 Fifteenth St., N.W., Washington, D.C., and is used by permission.

**Chapter 1: Understanding Your Sleep Connection**

1. Figures taken from the 1998 National Sleep Foundation Omnibus Sleep in America Poll.

**Chapter 2: Fixing a Faulty Sleep Connection**

1. Peter Hauri and Shirley Linde, *No More Sleepless Nights* (New York: John Wiley, 1991), p. 28.

**Chapter 3: The Mental Connection**

1. Taken from the 1998 National Sleep Foundation Omnibus Sleep in America Poll.

2. Hauri and Linde, *No More Sleepless Nights,* pp. 84-85.

**Chapter 4: The Physical Connection, Part 1**

1. Quote taken from the March 25, 1998 report on the 1998 National Sleep Foundation Omnibus Sleep in America Poll.

2. Benedict Carey, "The Slumber Solution," *Health* 10, no. 7 (1996): 72.

3. "Good Night, Asthma," *Prevention* 47, no. 5 (1995): 86.

4. Ibid., p. 88.

**Chapter 5: The Physical Connection, Part 2**

1. *Sleep Apnea* (Rochester, Minn.: American Sleep Disorders Association, 1992), p. 2.

2. Ibid., p. 82.

3. Taken from Jeanine Barone, "Fitful Slumber," *Better Homes and Gardens* 75, no. 7 (1997): 82.

4. For further information, contact the American Sleep Apnea Association, 2025 Pennsylvania Avenue NW, Suite 905, Washington, D.C. 20006; (202) 293-3650. This association promotes public awareness of sleep apnea, encourages research on the causes and treatments of breathing abnormalities during sleep, sponsors support groups for people with sleep apnea, and publishes a newsletter titled *Wake-Up Call.*

5. Margit Feury, "Sleep Apnea Warning," *Family Circle,* 19 November 1996, p. 58.

6. Samuel Dunkell, *Goodbye Insomnia, Hello Sleep* (New York: Dell Publishing, 1994), p. 162.

7. For more information, send a self-addressed stamped envelope to the Restless Legs Syndrome Foundation, 4410 19th Street NW, Suite 201, Rochester, MN 55901. This foundation provides educational information about RLS and works with an advisory board of doctors who specialize in neurological disorders. It publishes a bulletin and brochures, helps develop support groups, and provides information on research studies. Its Web site is http://www.rls.org.

8. Contact the Narcolepsy Network at P.O. Box 42460, Cincinnati, OH 45242; (513) 891-3522. This network educates the public about narcolepsy, helps establish support groups for narcoleptics and their families, and publishes educational brochures and a newsletter.

### Chapter 6: The Behavioral Connection

1. Diane Komp, *Breakfast for the Heart* (Grand Rapids, Mich.: Zondervan, 1996), p. 14.

### Chapter 7: The Day-Night Connection

1. *Circadian Rhythms: A Look at the Body's Natural Time Cues* (Rochester, Minn.: American Sleep Disorders Association, n.d.), p. 4.

2. Taken from a February 1997 newspaper article.

3. Carey, "The Slumber Solution," p. 74.

4. "Overcoming Insomnia," *Consumer Reports* 62, no. 3 (1997), p. 12.

5. "Shift Work and Poor Sleep: Permanent Bed Partners?" *The Shuteye News,* Winter 1996, p. 2.

### Chapter 8: The Environmental Connection

1. This survey, conducted September 13-15, 1996, by Bruskin/Golding Research for the Better Sleep Council, measured consumer awareness of four factors comprising the sleep environment: light, noise, temperature, and an uncomfortable mattress.

2. Quoted in Barbara Griggs, *Country Living's Healthy Living*: 52.

3. The Better Sleep Council, a nonprofit organization supported by the mattress industry, was established in 1978 to educate the public about "the importance of sleep to good health and quality of life and about the value of the sleep system and sleep environment in pursuit of a good night's sleep."

### Chapter 9: The Psychological Connection

1. Dunkell, *Goodbye Insomnia, Hello Sleep*, p. 11.

### Chapter 10: The Spiritual Connection

1. Tim Kimmel, *Little House on the Freeway: Help for the Hurried Home* (Sister, Or: Multnomah Press, 1994), p. 14.

2. Beginning is simply a matter of saying the "welcoming word to God—'Jesus is my Master'—embracing, body and soul, God's work of doing in us what he did in raising Jesus from the dead. That's it. You're not 'doing' anything; you're simply calling out to God, trusting him to do it for you. That's salvation. . . . Scripture reassures us, 'No one who trusts God like this—heart and soul—will ever regret it'" (Romans 10:9-11, *The Message*).

3. Linda K. DeVries, *Spiritual Nightlights: Meditations for the Middle of the Night* (Wheaton, Ill.: Harold Shaw Publishers, 1997), is available at your local Christian bookstore.

### Chapter 11: The Family Connection

1. Kimmel, *Little House on the Freeway*, p. 71.
2. Ibid.

### Chapter 13: The Professional Connection

1. Rosie Mestel, "Sleeping Lessons from Recovered Insomniacs," *Health* 11, no. 9 (1997): 110.

2. The American Sleep Disorders Association (ASDA), founded in 1987, is a professional medical association that represents practitioners of sleep medicine and sleep research. For a list of

sleep disorder centers near you, write to the ASDA, 1610 14th Street NW, Suite 300, Rochester, MN 55901 or visit their Web site at http://www.asda.org.

## Appendix A: What You Should Know about Medications and Health Remedies

1. This list was compiled from information in Hauri and Linde, *No More Sleepless Nights,* pp. 165-166, and Charles M. Morin, *Relief from Insomnia* (New York: Doubleday, 1996), pp. 36-37.

2. David J. Kupfer and Charles F. Reynolds III, "Management of Insomnia," *The New England Journal of Medicine* 336, no. 5 (1997): 342.

3. Mestel, "Sleeping Lessons from Recovered Insomniacs," p. 115.

4. Kupfer and Reynolds, "Management of Insomnia," p. 345.

5. Mestel, "Sleeping Lessons from Recovered Insomniacs," p. 115.

6. W. Gifford-Jones, "Vitamin E Can Help Get the Kinks Out," *The Post-Crescent* newspaper, Appleton, Wisconsin, 29 April 1995.

# Bibliography

## Books

Dotto, Lydia. *Losing Sleep: How Your Sleeping Habits Affect Your Life*. New York: William Morrow & Co., 1990.

Dunkell, Samuel. *Goodbye Insomnia, Hello Sleep*. New York: Dell Publishing, 1994.

Ford, Norman. *The Sleep Rx*. New York: Prentice-Hall, 1994.

Hauri, Peter, and Shirley Linde. *No More Sleepless Nights*. New York: John Wiley and Sons, 1991.

*International Classification of Sleep Disorders*. Rochester, Minn.: American Sleep Disorders Association, 1990.

Kimmel, Tim. *Little House on the Freeway: Help for the Hurried Home*. Sisters, Ore.: Multnomah, 1994.

Kryger, Meir, Thomas Roth, and William C. Dement, eds. *Principles and Practice of Sleep Medicine*. 2nd ed. Philadelphia, Penn.: W.B. Saunders, 1994.

Lavie, Peretz. *The Enchanted World of Sleep*. New Haven, Conn.: Yale University Press, 1996.

Mitler, Elizabeth A., and Merrill M. Mitler. *101 Questions About Sleep and Dreams*. 4th ed. Del Mar, Calif.: Wakefulness-Sleep Education and Research Foundation, 1993.

Morin, Charles M. *Relief from Insomnia: Getting the Sleep of Your Dreams*. New York: Doubleday, 1996.

Soth, Connie. *Insomnia: God's Night School*. Old Tappan, N.J.: Fleming H. Revell, 1989.

## Pamphlets/Brochures

*The Better Sleep Guide*. Alexandria, Va.: The Better Sleep Council, 1996.

*Circadian Rhythms: A Look at the Body's Natural Time Cues*. Rochester, Minn.: American Sleep Disorders Association, n.d.

*Coping with Shift Work.* Alexandria, Va.: The Better Sleep Council, 1994.

*Insomnia.* Rochester, Minn.: American Sleep Disorders Association, 1992.

*Parasomnias: Things That Go Bump in the Night.* Rochester, Minn.: American Sleep Disorders Association, 1994.

*Restless Legs Syndrome and Periodic Limb Movement Disorder.* Rochester, Minn.: American Sleep Disorders Association, 1994.

*Sleep As We Grow Older.* Rochester, Minn.: American Sleep Disorders Association, 1994.

## Articles

Barone, Jeanine. "Fitful Slumber." *Better Homes and Gardens* 75, no. 7 (1997): 80-84.

Carey, Benedict, and Kate Lee. "The Slumber Solution." *Health* 10, no. 4 (1996): 71-74.

Eberlein, Tamara. "Getting Bedtime Right." *Working Mother* 19, no. 9 (1996): 41-44.

Feury, Margit. "Sleep Apnea Warning." *Family Circle* (19 November 1996): 58.

Field, David. "Sleep-Tight Room Renders Reporter a Shell of a Man." *USA Today* (25 March 1997): 5E.

Foster, Stephen. " 'Perchance to Dream . . . ?' Herbs to Help Us Sleep." *Better Nutrition* 59, no. 3 (1997): 64-68.

Geier, Thom. "What Is Sleep For?" *U.S. News and World Report* (18-25 August 1997): 48-51.

"Good Night, Asthma." *Prevention* 46, no. 5 (1995): 86-90.

Gower, Timothy. "America's Hidden Health Crisis." *The Walking Magazine* 12, no. 5 (1997): 50-8.

Hall, Stephen S. "Cures by the Clock." *Health* 10, no. 4 (1996): 106-8.

Hall, Susan Bard. "Hilton Program Helps Provide Rest for Weary Guests." *Hotel and Motel Management* (17 February 1997).

Hauri, Peter J. "Consulting About Insomnia: A Method and Some Preliminary Data." *Sleep* 16, no. 4 (1993): 344-50.

Hutter, Sarah. "Is Your Child Getting Enough Sleep?" *Woman's Day* (1 February 1995): 38-40.

Johnson, Kathleen. "The Best (and Worst) Late-Night Snacks." *The Well Street Review* (Winter 1995): 5.

# Bibliography

King, Abby C., Roy F. Oman, Glenn S. Brassington, Donald L. Bliwise, and William L. Haskell. "Moderate-Intensity Exercise and Self-Rated Qualities of Sleep in Older Adults: A Randomized Controlled Trial." *Journal of the American Medical Association* 277, no. 1 (Jan 1,1997): 32-37.

Klinkenborg, Verlyn. "Awakening to Sleep." *The New York Times Magazine* (5 January 1997), sec. 6:26+.

Kupfer, David J. and Charles F. Reynolds. "Management of Insomnia." *New England Journal of Medicine* 336, no. 5 (1997): 341-6.

Laliberte, Richard. "Are Sleep Robbers Stealing Your Zzzzs?" *McCall's* 123, no. 8 (May 1996): 90-92.

Legwold, Gary. "Emotions and Your Health." *Better Homes and Gardens* 72, no. 10 (1994): 60.

Mestel, Rosie. "Sleeping Lessons from Recovered Insomniacs." *Health* 11, no. 9 (1997): 109-115.

Meyer, Michele. "Laughter: It's Good Medicine." *Better Homes and Gardens* 75, no. 4 (1997): 72-6.

Murphy, Caryle. "Researchers Urge Skepticism on Melatonin." *Washington Post* 119, no. 259 (1996): WH7, col. 1.

"The National Sleep Debt," *USA Weekend* (3-5 January 1997): 4-24.

"NIH Releases Statement on Behavioral and Relaxation Approaches for Chronic Pain and Insomnia." *American Family Physician* 53, no. 5 (1996): 1877-9.

"Overcoming Insomnia." *Consumer Reports* 62, no. 3 (1997): 10-13.

"Overcoming Insomnia." *Mayo Clinic Health Letter* 14, no. 11 (1996): 3.

"Relief for Window Rattlers." *Kiplinger's Personal Finance Magazine* 50, no. 7 (July 1996): 94.

Seal, Kathy. "Hilton Tests Sleep Aids Chainwide." *Hotel and Motel Management* (22 July 1996).

"Shift Work and Poor Sleep: Permanent Bed Partners?" *The Shuteye News* (Winter 1996): 2.

"Silent Cause of Traffic Deaths: Falling Asleep." *USA Weekend* (16-19 May 1997): 12.

Tonnessen, Diana. "The Family Bed: Should You Allow Your Child to Sleep with You?" *Parents Magazine* 71, no. 7 (1996): 47-8.

# Index

Adolescents, sleep needs of, 22, 125, 155

Adults, sleep needs of, 43, 50; (*see also* Men; Older adults; Women)

Advanced sleep phase syndrome, 92

Alcohol and insomnia, 25, 26, 29, 31, 35, 61, 68, 80, 89

Allergies, 30, 54-55, 56, 79

American Sleep Disorders Association, 19, 91, 144, 147, 156

Anger, 54, 68, 104, 110-111

Antidepressant medications, 63, 65, 70, 130, 149, 151

Antihistamines, 55, 151

Anxiety, role in insomnia, 32, 33, 66, 68, 100, 105-106, 116, 143, 151

Apnea, *see* Sleep apnea

Asthma, 55-56

Attitudes, toward sleep, 14, 35, 37-46, 143

Bedrooms, 67, 92, 95-101, 124, 126, 138

Beds, 25, 42, 92, 96-98, 124

Bedtime routines, 28, 44, 71, 75, 82, 122, 137; (*see also* Habits)

Bed-wetting, 61, 128-130

Behavior therapies for insomnia, 66, 71-83

Bible references, 38, 53, 82, 101, 102, 107, 114, 116-117

Body clock, 14, 55, 84-94, 125, 126, 156

Brain waves, 16-18, 60, 67, 69

Breathing, 40, 73
    problems, 25, 26, 30, 48, 49, 54, 58-61, 145, 148, 151; (*see also* Sleep apnea)

Caffeine, 25, 29, 31, 34, 35, 44, 64, 79, 80, 92, 102, 131, 146, 151

Calcium, 65, 154

Central sleep apnea, 60-61

Children, sleep needs, 44, 61, 62, 63, 119-132, 157

Chronic insomnia, *see* Insomnia

Circadian rhythms, 26, 84-94; (*see also* Body clock)

Clock, alarm, 100-101, 137

Cognitive therapy, changing beliefs and attitudes, 40, 43, 45

Conditioned insomnia, 42

Continuous positive airway pressure (CPAP), 60, 148

Counseling, *see* Psychiatric counseling

Cycles, sleep, *see* Body clock; Sleep cycles

Day-night cycles, 28, 84-86, 99, 155

Daytime sleepiness, 19, 27, 58, 59, 64, 68, 121, 147

Deep sleep, 18, 50, 51, 80, 150, 155

Delayed sleep phase syndrome, 92, 126

Depression, 25, 26, 27, 32-34, 59, 104, 109-110, 111, 125, 143, 151

Diet/nutrition, 64, 65, 77-79, 89, 135, 153, 154

Dopamine, 63, 150

Elderly, *see* Older adults

Electroencephalograph (EEG), 16, 18, 69

Emotions, insomnia and, 32-34, 104-111, 136; (*see also* Anxiety; Depression; Stress),

Environment, effect on sleep, 25, 26, 35, 95-103, 125, 138

Exercise, 35, 51, 65, 71-72, 82, 89, 130, 135

Faith (trust), 37, 54, 114-115

Fatigue, 19, 47, 73, 76, 83, 91

Fear, 15, 25, 45, 104, 106-108, 123, 134

# Index

(Fear cont.)
  of insomnia, 35, 37, 41-42, 44, 140, 148
Frequent waking, 23, 26, 27, 58, 80, 81, 119, 121

Gender differences, sleep, 48-50, 59, 65, 67, 127, 128
GHB (Gamma hydroxybutyrate), 154-155
Grief, 25, 26, 104, 108-109, 132

Habits, sleep-related, 25, 28, 44, 48, 118-120, 121, 122-124, 134, 137
Herbal remedies, 151-153
Heredity, 63, 69, 85, 127
History, sleep, 27-28
Hormones, and sleep, 18, 48, 49, 55, 85, 93, 150, 155

Illness and sleep, 25, 30-31, 51-53, 132-133
Infants, 22, 48, 61, 94, 119-122
Insomnia,
  causes of, 24-25, 30-36, 104-111
  childhood-onset, 130
  chronic, 19-20, 26, 51, 151
  conditioned, 42
  effects of, 19-21
  fear of, 35, 37, 41-42, 44, 140
  prevalence, 13, 38, 104
  temporary (transient), 19, 25-26, 150
  types of, 25-26
  (see also Medical Causes; Physical Factors; Physicians)

Jet lag, 25, 88-90, 93, 150, 155
Journal/writing, 28, 36, 43, 45, 53, 106, 109, 116, 117

Leg cramps, see Nocturnal leg cramps; Periodic limb movements; Restless legs syndrome
Lifestyle, effects on sleep, 34-36, 71-83, 135, 152
Light, 84-86, 89, 92, 94, 99, 124, 130, 153
  therapy, 85-86, 89, 92, 93
Light-dark cycle, 84-86, 99, 124

Marriage partners, and sleep disruptions, 61, 131-141
Massage, therapeutic, 53, 64, 66, 76-77, 135

Medical causes of insomnia, 30-31, 47-56, 132-133
Medications,
  causing insomnia, 25, 26, 31, 56, 64, 133, 149-150
  to treat insomnia, 52, 63, 65, 66, 67, 69, 106, 128, 130, 143, 150-151
  (see also Antidepressant medications; Sleeping pills)
Melatonin, 90, 93-94, 155
Men, and sleep, 48, 50, 59, 65, 67
Menopause, 25, 48, 49, 59

Napping, 27, 29, 42, 69, 86-87, 88, 121
Narcolepsy, 68-70, 125, 147, 155, 156
National Sleep Foundation, 13, 102, 157, 159
Nicotine, and insomnia, 35, 80-81
Nightmares, 30, 127-128
Nocturnal leg cramps, 65-66, 154
Noise, 73-74, 92, 95, 99-100, 102, 153
Non-drug therapies, 151-155
Non-rapid eye movement sleep (NREM), see Sleep

Obstructive sleep apnea, see Sleep apnea
Older adults, 48, 60-61, 63, 67, 155
  sleep patterns of, 18, 22-23, 50-51

Pain, and sleep, 25, 26, 30, 51-53, 74, 98, 149
Periodic limb movements (PLM), 49, 64-65
Phase delay insomnia, 92-93, 125
Physical factors, affecting sleep, 30-31, 47-56, 57-70, 128, 143
Physicians, insomnia treatment by, 28, 30, 42, 47, 52, 54, 60, 63, 70, 74, 86-87, 96, 106, 125, 129-130, 140-141, 142-143, 147, 149; (see also Sleep clinics; Sleep specialists; Psychiatric counseling)
Polysomnography, 60, 69, 146-147
Prayer, 40, 53-54, 106, 109, 115-116, 136
Pregnancy, 49, 63, 65, 66, 94, 98
Psychiatric counseling, 68, 106, 109, 110, 128, 141, 143
Psychological causes, 32-34, 104-112, 126; (see also Anger; Anxiety; Depression; Fear; Grief; Stress)

# Index

Questionnaires, 27-35

Rapid eye movement sleep (REM),
    see Sleep
Relaxation, 43-44, 72-74, 154
REM-sleep behavior disorder, 18, 67
Rest, 15, 16, 62-64, 106, 108
    spiritual, 54, 106, 112-117
Restless legs syndrome (RLS), 62-64,
    154, 157, 160

Security of sleep environment, 101,
    134
Serotonin, 151, 154
Sexual relations, 124, 135, 138
Shift work, 14, 20, 25, 27, 90-92
Short-term insomnia, 25, 26
Sleep,
    changes with age, 18, 22-23, 26,
        50-51,
    cycles, 16-18, 84-94
    debt (deprivation, loss), 13,
        19-21, 50, 126
    definition, 16
    NREM, 16-18, 68
    patterns (schedules, rhythms), 15,
        27, 28, 41-42, 49, 50-52, 68, 80,
        84-85, 87-94, 125, 143, 149
    quantity (needs), 16, 21-22, 29,
        50, 120-121
    REM, 16-18, 67, 68, 127
    stages, 16-18
Sleep apnea, obstructive, 57-61, 62,
    80, 156
Sleep clinics/disorders centers,
    143-147, 158, 162
Sleep disorders, 57-70, 93, 156-158;
    (see also specific disorders)

Sleep journal, see Journal
Sleep specialists, 29-30, 31, 39, 70,
    87, 143, 147
Sleep terrors, 126-127
Sleeping pills, 25, 31, 80, 92, 130,
    141, 150-151
Sleepwalking, 31, 66, 126
Smoking, see Nicotine
Snoring, 30, 59, 61-62, 144
Spiritual rest, see Rest
Spouses, and sleep, 61, 132-142
Stress (tension),
    effects of, 25, 32, 34, 91,
        104-105, 127, 128, 133
    managing, 34-35, 68, 71-77, 131,
        152
Sudden infant death syndrome
    (SIDS), 48, 61
Sunday night insomnia, 88
Support groups, 53, 70, 139, 158,
    160

Teenagers, see Adolescents
Temperature,
    body, 18, 50, 85, 120
    room, 95, 98-99
Tooth-grinding (bruxism), 30, 68
Tranquilizers, 61, 66, 150
Transient insomnia, 19, 25-26,
    151-152
Tryptophan, 78, 154

Vitamins and minerals, 65-66,
    153-154

Women, and sleep, 48-49, 59, 65
Worry, 33, 44, 104-106, 140; (see
    also Anxiety)